£25.00

RADIATION PROTECTION

1990 Recommendations of the International Commission on Radiological Protection

ADOPTED BY THE COMMISSION IN NOVEMBER 1990

Users' Edition

PUBLISHED FOR

The International Commission on Radiological Protection

by

PERGAMON PRESS

OXFORD · NEW YORK · SEOUL · TOKYO

UK   Pergamon Press Ltd, Headington Hill Hall,
Oxford OX3 0BW, England

USA   Pergamon Press Inc., 660 White Plains Road, Tarrytown,
NY 10591-5153, USA

KOREA   Pergamon Press Korea, Room 613 Hanaro Building,
194-4 Insa-Dong, Chongno-ku, Seoul 110-290, Korea

JAPAN   Pergamon Press, Tsunashima Building Annex, 3-20-12 Yushima,
Bunkyo-ku, Tokyo 113, Japan

First edition 1992
ISBN 0 08 041998 4
ISSN 0146-6453

*Typeset by Cotswold Typesetting Ltd, Gloucester
Printed and bound in Great Britain by BPCC Wheatons Ltd,
Exeter*

CONTENTS

The annexes have been omitted from this edition

PREFACE TO THE USERS' EDITION OF THE 1990 RECOMMENDATIONS OF THE INTERNATIONAL COMMISSION ON RADIOLOGICAL PROTECTION

This "Users' Edition" of the Commission's 1990 Recommendations contains in full the main text of the recommendations, but excludes the four annexes. The text has been provided with a more comprehensive index. It is aimed at individual users in both regulatory and operational organisations who need frequent access to the Recommendations, but have only an occasional need to consult the annexes.

The complete text with the annexes, now called the "Reference Edition", is still available as *ICRP Publication 60, Annals of the ICRP*, Volume 21 No. 1–3. Any references in the Users' Edition to annexes relate to those in the Reference Edition.

PREFACE

(1) Since 1977, when the Commission issued its basic recommendations as *ICRP Publication 26*, it has reviewed these recommendations annually and, from time to time, has issued supplementary Statements in the *Annals of the ICRP*. A complete list of the Commission's publications is given in Annex D. Developments in the last few years have now made it necessary to issue a completely new set of recommendations. In doing so, the Commission has had three aims in mind:

(a) to take account of new biological information and of trends in the setting of safety standards,
(b) to improve the presentation of the recommendations,
(c) to maintain as much stability in the recommendations as is consistent with the new information.

(2) The draft of these recommendations was prepared by a Task Group set up by the 1985–89 Commission and comprising:

D. Beninson (Chairman)	Chairman of the Commission
H. Jammet	Vice-Chairman of the Commission
W. K. Sinclair	Chairman of Committee 1
C. B. Meinhold	Chairman of Committee 2
J. Liniecki	Chairman of Committee 3
H. J. Dunster	Chairman of Committee 4 to 1989
R. H. Clarke	Chairman of Committee 4 from 1989
B. Lindell	Emeritus Member of the Commission
H. Smith (Secretary)	Scientific Secretary of the Commission

The draft was discussed and adopted by the 1989–93 Commission in November 1990.

COMMISSION MEMBERSHIP, 1985–89		COMMISSION MEMBERSHIP, 1989–93	
D. Beninson	Chairman	D. Beninson	Chairman
H. Jammet	Vice-Chairman	H. Jammet	Vice-Chairman
R. J. Berry		R. H. Clarke	Chairman, Committee 4
H. J. Dunster	Chairman, Committee 4	H. J. Dunster	
W. Jacobi		A. K. Guskova	
D. Li		W. Jacobi	
J. Liniecki	Chairman, Committee 3	D. Li	
C. B. Meinhold	Chairman, Committee 2	J. Liniecki	Chairman, Committee 3
A. K. Poznanski		C. B. Meinhold	Chairman, Committee 2
P. V. Ramzaev		F. Mettler	
G. Silini		I. Shigematsu	
W. K. Sinclair	Chairman, Committee 1	G. Silini	
E. Tajima		W. K. Sinclair	Chairman, Committee 1
H. Smith	Scientific Secretary	H. Smith	Scientific Secretary

1. INTRODUCTION

Chapter 1 deals with the history of the Commission and its recommendations. It sets out the aims and form of this report. It indicates why the Commission concerns itself only with the protection of man and only with ionising radiation. A list of the Publications of the Commission is given in Annex D.

1.1. The History of the Commission

(3) The International Commission on Radiological Protection, hereafter called the Commission, was established in 1928, with the name of the International X ray and Radium Protection Committee, following a decision by the Second International Congress of Radiology. In 1950 it was restructured and renamed. The Commission still retains a special relationship with the four-yearly Congress meetings and with the International Society of Radiology but, over the years, has greatly broadened its interests to take account of the increasing uses of ionising radiation and of practices that involve the generation of radiation and radioactive materials.

(4) The Commission works closely with its sister body, the International Commission on Radiation Units and Measurements, and has official relationships with the World Health Organisation and the International Atomic Energy Agency. It also has important relationships with the International Labour Organisation and other United Nations bodies, including the United Nations Scientific Committee on the Effects of Atomic Radiation and the United Nations Environment Programme, and with the Commission of the European Communities, the Nuclear Energy Agency of the Organisation for Economic Co-operation and Development, the International Standards Organisation, the International Electrotechnical Commission, and the International Radiation Protection Association. It takes account of progress reported by major national organisations.

(5) The Commission issued its first report in 1928. The first report in the current series, subsequently numbered *Publication 1* (1959), contained the recommendations approved in September 1958. Subsequent general recommendations have appeared as *Publication 6* (1964), *Publication 9* (1966), and *Publication 26* (1977). *Publication 26* was amended and extended by a Statement in 1978 and further clarified and extended by Statements in later years (1980, 1983, 1984, 1985, and 1987). Reports on more specialised topics have appeared as intermediate and subsequent publication numbers (Annex D).

1.2. The Development of the Commission's Recommendations

(6) The method of working of the Commission has not changed greatly over the last few decades. Since there is little direct evidence of harm at levels of annual dose at or below the limits recommended by the Commission, a good deal of scientific judgement is required in predicting the probability of harm resulting from low doses. Most of the observed data have been obtained at higher doses and usually at high dose rates. The Commission's aim is to draw on a broad spectrum of expertise from outside sources as well as from its own Committees and Task Groups and thus to reach a reasonable consensus about the outcome of exposures to radiation. It has not thought it appropriate

to use either the most pessimistic or the most optimistic interpretation of the available data, but has aimed at using estimates that are not likely to underestimate the consequences of exposures. The estimation of these consequences and their implications necessarily involves social and economic judgements as well as scientific judgements in a wide range of disciplines. The Commission has aimed to make the basis of such judgements as clear as possible, and recognises that others may wish to reach their own conclusions on many of the issues.

(7) The Commission has found that its recommendations have been used both by regulatory authorities and by management bodies and their specialist advisers. Because of the wide range of situations to which the Commission's recommendations might be applied, the degree of detail has deliberately been restricted. However, the Commission has had historical links with medical radiology and its advice in this area has often been more detailed.

(8) The Commission's recommendations have helped to provide a consistent basis for national and regional regulatory standards. For its part, the Commission has been concerned to maintain stability in its recommendations. It believes that frequent changes would only cause confusion. The Commission reviews the newly published data annually against the background of the much larger accumulation of existing data. It is not likely that dramatic changes would be called for by these reviews, but if new data should show the existing recommendations to be in need of urgent change, the Commission would respond rapidly.

(9) Over the last few decades, there has been a significant change in emphasis in the presentation and application of the system of protection recommended by the Commission. Initially, and into the 1950s, there was a tendency to regard compliance with the limits on individual doses as being a measure of satisfactory achievement. The advice that all exposures should be kept as low as possible was noted, but not often applied consciously. Since then, much more emphasis has been put on the requirement to keep all exposures "as low as reasonably achievable, economic and social factors being taken into account". This emphasis has resulted in substantial decreases in individual doses and has greatly reduced the number of situations in which the dose limits play a major role in the overall system of protection. It has also changed the purpose of the dose limits recommended by the Commission. Initially, their main function was the avoidance of directly observable, non-malignant effects. Subsequently, they were also intended to limit the incidence of cancer and hereditary effects caused by radiation. Over the years, the limits have been expressed in a variety of ways, so that comparisons are not easy. In broad terms, however, the annual limit for occupational exposure of the whole body was reduced by a factor of about 3 between 1934 and 1950, and by a further factor of 3, to the equivalent of 50 mSv, by 1958.

1.3. The Aims of this Report

(10) The Commission intends this report to be of help to regulatory and advisory agencies at national, regional, and international levels, mainly by providing guidance on the fundamental principles on which appropriate radiological protection can be based. Because of the differing conditions that apply in various countries, the Commission does not intend to provide a regulatory text. Authorities will need to develop their own structures of legislation, regulation, authorisations, licences, codes of practice, and guidance material in line with their usual practices and policies. The Commission

believes that these regulatory structures should be designed to be broadly consistent with the guidancé in this report. In addition, the Commission hopes that the report will be of help to management bodies with responsibilities for radiological protection in their own operations, to the professional staff whom they use as their advisers, and to individuals, such as radiologists, who have to make decisions about the use of ionising radiation.

(11) The Commission has therefore set out these recommendations in the form of a main text supported by more detailed annexes. The main text contains all the recommendations, together with sufficient explanatory material to make clear the underlying reasoning. It is intended to be used by those concerned with policy, who can turn to the supporting annexes if they need more detailed information on specific points. Specialists will need to study both the main text and the annexes.

(12) Chapters 2 and 3 deal with the quantities and units used in radiological protection and with the biological effects of radiation. Chapter 4 describes the conceptual framework of radiological protection and leads into Chapters 5 and 6 which deal with the Commission's main recommendations. Chapter 7 discusses the practical implementation of the recommendations. Finally, there is a summary of the recommendations.

1.4. The Scope of the Commission's Recommendations

(13) Ionisation is the process by which atoms lose, or sometimes gain electrons and thus become electrically charged, being then known as ions. Ionising radiation is the term used to describe the transfer of energy through space in the form of either electromagnetic waves or subatomic particles that are capable of causing ionisation in matter. When ionising radiation passes through matter, energy is imparted to the matter as ions are formed.

(14) The recommendations of the Commission, as in previous reports, are confined to protection against ionising radiation. The Commission recognises the importance of adequate control over sources of non-ionising radiation, but continues to consider that this is a subject outside its own field of competence. It also recognises that this concentration on a single one of the many dangers facing mankind may cause an unwanted element of anxiety. The Commission therefore wishes to emphasise its view that ionising radiation needs to be treated with care rather than fear and that its risks should be kept in perspective with other risks. The procedures available to control exposures to ionising radiation are sufficient, if used properly, to ensure that it remains a minor component of the spectrum of risks to which we are all exposed.

(15) Ionising radiation and radioactive materials have always been features of our environment, but, owing to their lack of impact on our senses, we became aware of them only at the end of the 19th century. Since that time, we have found many important uses for them and have developed new technological processes which create them, either deliberately or as unwanted by-products. The primary aim of radiological protection is to provide an appropriate standard of protection for man without unduly limiting the beneficial practices giving rise to radiation exposure. This aim cannot be achieved on the basis of scientific concepts alone. All those concerned with radiological protection have to make value judgements about the relative importance of different kinds of risk and about the balancing of risks and benefits. In this, they are no different from those working in other fields concerned with the control of hazards.

(16) The Commission believes that the standard of environmental control needed to protect man to the degree currently thought desirable will ensure that other species are

not put at risk. Occasionally, individual members of non-human species might be harmed, but not to the extent of endangering whole species or creating imbalance between species. At the present time, the Commission concerns itself with mankind's environment only with regard to the transfer of radionuclides through the environment, since this directly affects the radiological protection of man.

2. QUANTITIES USED IN RADIOLOGICAL PROTECTION

Chapter 2 explains in simple terms the principal quantities used in radiological protection. The formal definitions and more detailed information are given in Annex A.

2.1. Introduction

(17) Historically, the quantities used to measure the "amount" of ionising radiation (subsequently called "radiation" in this report) have been based on the gross number of ionising events in a defined situation or on the gross amount of energy deposited, usually in a defined mass of material. These approaches omit consideration of the discontinuous nature of the process of ionisation, but are justified empirically by the observation that the gross quantities (with adjustments for different types of radiation) correlate fairly well with the resulting biological effects.

(18) Future developments may well show that it would be better to use other quantities based on the statistical distribution of events in a small volume of material corresponding to the dimensions of biological entities such as the nucleus of the cell or its molecular DNA. Meanwhile, however, the Commission continues to recommend the use of macroscopic quantities. These, among others, are described in Annex A and are known as dosimetric quantities. They have been defined in formal terms by the International Commission on Radiation Units and Measurements (ICRU).

(19) Before discussing dosimetric quantities, it is necessary to anticipate some of the information on the biological effects of radiation described in Chapter 3. The process of ionisation necessarily changes atoms and molecules, at least transiently, and may thus sometimes damage cells. If cellular damage does occur, and is not adequately repaired, it may prevent the cell from surviving or reproducing, or it may result in a viable but modified cell. The two outcomes have profoundly different implications for the organism as a whole.

(20) Most organs and tissues of the body are unaffected by the loss of even substantial numbers of cells, but if the number lost is large enough, there will be observable harm reflecting a loss of tissue function. The probability of causing such harm will be zero at small doses, but above some level of dose (the threshold) will increase steeply to unity (100%). Above the threshold, the severity of the harm will also increase with dose. For reasons explained in Section 3.4.1, this type of effect, previously called "non-stochastic", is now called "deterministic" by the Commission.

(21) The outcome is very different if the irradiated cell is modified rather than killed. Despite the existence of highly effective defence mechanisms, the clone of cells resulting from the reproduction of a modified but viable somatic cell may result, after a prolonged and variable delay called the latency period, in the manifestation of a malignant condition, a cancer. The probability of a cancer resulting from radiation usually increases with increments of dose, probably with no threshold, and in a way that is roughly proportional to dose, at least for doses well below the thresholds for deterministic effects. The

severity of the cancer is not affected by the dose. This kind of effect is called "stochastic", meaning "of a random or statistical nature". If the damage occurs in a cell whose function is to transmit genetic information to later generations, any resulting effects, which may be of many different kinds and severity, are expressed in the progeny of the exposed person. This type of stochastic effect is called "hereditary".

2.2. Basic Dosimetric Quantities

(22) The fundamental dosimetric quantity in radiological protection is the **absorbed dose**, D. This is the energy absorbed per unit mass and its unit is the joule per kilogram, which is given the special name gray (Gy). Absorbed dose is defined in terms that allow it to be specified at a point, but it is used in this report, except where otherwise stated, to mean the average dose over a tissue or organ. The use of the average dose as an indicator of the probability of subsequent stochastic effects depends on the linearity of the relationship between the probability of inducing an effect and the dose (the dose–response relationship)—a reasonable approximation over a limited range of dose. The dose–response relationship is not linear for deterministic effects so the average absorbed dose is not directly relevant to deterministic effects unless the dose is fairly uniformly distributed over the tissue or organ.

2.2.1. Radiation weighting factors

(23) The probability of stochastic effects is found to depend, not only on the absorbed dose, but also on the type and energy of the radiation causing the dose. This is taken into account by weighting the absorbed dose by a factor related to the quality of the radiation. In the past, this weighting factor has been applied to the absorbed dose at a point and called the quality factor, Q. The weighted absorbed dose was called the dose equivalent, H.

2.2.2. Equivalent dose

(24) In radiological protection, it is the absorbed dose averaged over a tissue or organ (rather than at a point) and weighted for the radiation quality that is of interest. The weighting factor for this purpose is now called the **radiation weighting factor**, w_R, and is selected for the type and energy of the radiation incident on the body or, in the case of sources within the body, emitted by the source. This weighted absorbed dose is strictly a dose, and the Commission has decided to revert to the earlier name of **equivalent dose** in a tissue or organ, using the symbol H_T. The change of name also serves to indicate the change from quality factor to radiation weighting factor. The equivalent dose in tissue T is given by the expression

$$H_T = \sum_R w_R \cdot D_{T,R}$$

where $D_{T,R}$ is the absorbed dose averaged over the tissue or organ T, due to radiation R. The unit of equivalent dose is the joule per kilogram with the special name sievert (Sv).

(25) The value of the radiation weighting factor for a specified type and energy of radiation has been selected by the Commission to be representative of values of the relative biological effectiveness of that radiation in inducing stochastic effects at low doses. The **relative biological effectiveness** (RBE) of one radiation compared with another is the inverse ratio of the absorbed doses producing the same degree of a defined

biological end-point. The values of w_R are broadly compatible with the values of Q, which are related to the quantity linear energy transfer (LET), a measure of the density of ionisation along the track of an ionising particle. This relationship was originally intended to do no more than provide a rough indication of the variation of the values of Q with changes of radiation, but it was often interpreted to imply a spurious precision which the Commission hopes will not be inferred from the new radiation weighting factors. The Commission has chosen a value of radiation weighting factor of unity for all radiations of low LET, including x and gamma radiations of all energies. The choice for other radiations is based on observed values of the relative biological effectiveness (RBE), regardless of whether the reference radiation is x or gamma radiation.

(26) When the radiation field is composed of types and energies with different values of w_R, the absorbed dose must be subdivided in blocks, each with its own value of w_R and summed to give the total equivalent dose. Alternatively it may be expressed as a continuous distribution in energy where each element of absorbed dose from the energy element between E and $E + dE$ is multiplied by the value of w_R from the relevant block in Table 1 or, as an approximation, by the value of w_R from the continuous function given in paragraph A12 of Annex A and illustrated by the continuous curve in Figure 1. The basis for selecting values for other radiations is given in Annex A (paragraph A13). Auger electrons emitted from nuclei bound to DNA present a special problem because it is not realistic to average the absorbed dose over the whole mass of DNA as would be required by the present definition of equivalent dose. The effects of Auger electrons have to be assessed by the techniques of microdosimetry (see Annex B, paragraph B67).

Table 1. Radiation weighting factors[1]

Type and energy range[2]	Radiation weighting factor, w_R
Photons, all energies	1
Electrons and muons, all energies[3]	1
Neutrons, energy < 10 keV	5
10 keV to 100 keV	10
> 100 keV to 2 MeV	20
> 2 MeV to 20 MeV	10
> 20 MeV	5
(See also Figure 1)	
Protons, other than recoil protons, energy > 2 MeV	5
Alpha particles, fission fragments, heavy nuclei	20

[1] All values relate to the radiation incident on the body or, for internal sources, emitted from the source.

[2] The choice of values for other radiations is discussed in Annex A.

[3] Excluding Auger electrons emitted from nuclei bound to DNA (see paragraph 26).

2.2.3. *Tissue weighting factors and effective dose*

(27) The relationship between the probability of stochastic effects and equivalent dose is found also to depend on the organ or tissue irradiated. It is therefore appropriate to define a further quantity, derived from equivalent dose, to indicate the combination of different doses to several different tissues in a way which is likely to correlate well with the total of the stochastic effects. The factor by which the equivalent dose in tissue or organ T is weighted is called the **tissue weighting factor**, w_T which represents the relative

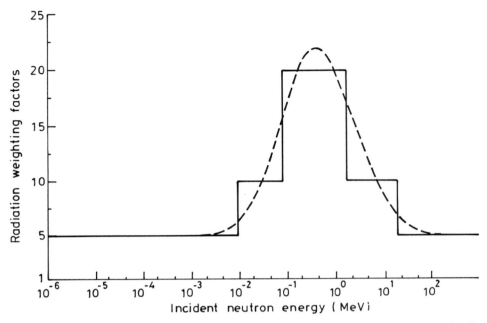

Fig. 1. Radiation weighting factors for neutrons. The smooth curve is to be treated as an approximation.

contribution of that organ or tissue to the total detriment due to these effects resulting from uniform irradiation of the whole body. (See Section 3.5.) The weighted equivalent dose (a doubly weighted absorbed dose) has previously been called the effective dose equivalent but this name is unnecessarily cumbersome, especially in more complex combinations such as collective committed effective dose equivalent. The Commission has now decided to use the simpler name **effective dose**, E. The introduction of the name effective dose is associated with the change to equivalent dose, but has no connection with changes in the number or magnitude of the tissue weighting factors. The unit is the joule per kilogram with the special name sievert. The choice of values of the tissue weighting factor is discussed in Section 3.5 and the recommended values are given in Table 2.

(28) The effective dose is the sum of the weighted equivalent doses in all the tissues and organs of the body. It is given by the expression

$$E = \sum_{T} w_T \cdot H_T$$

where H_T is the equivalent dose in tissue or organ T and w_T is the weighting factor for tissue T. The effective dose can also be expressed as the sum of the doubly weighted absorbed dose in all the tissues and organs of the body.

(29) It is desirable that a uniform equivalent dose over the whole body should give an effective dose numerically equal to that uniform equivalent dose. This is achieved by normalising the sum of the tissue weighting factors to unity. The values of the radiation weighting factor depend on the type and energy of the radiation and are independent of the tissue or organ. Similarly, the values of the tissue weighting factor are chosen to be independent of the type and energy of the radiation incident on the body. These simplifi-

Table 2. Tissue weighting factors[1]

Tissue or organ	Tissue weighting factor, w_T
Gonads	0.20
Bone marrow (red)	0.12
Colon	0.12
Lung	0.12
Stomach	0.12
Bladder	0.05
Breast	0.05
Liver	0.05
Oesophagus	0.05
Thyroid	0.05
Skin	0.01
Bone surface	0.01
Remainder	0.05[2,3]

[1] The values have been developed from a reference population of equal numbers of both sexes and a wide range of ages. In the definition of effective dose they apply to workers, to the whole population, and to either sex.

[2] For purposes of calculation, the remainder is composed of the following additional tissues and organs: adrenals, brain, upper large intestine, small intestine, kidney, muscle, pancreas, spleen, thymus and uterus. The list includes organs which are likely to be selectively irradiated. Some organs in the list are known to be susceptible to cancer induction. If other tissues and organs subsequently become identified as having a significant risk of induced cancer they will then be included either with a specific w_T or in this additional list constituting the remainder. The latter may also include other tissues or organs selectively irradiated.

[3] In those exceptional cases in which a single one of the remainder tissues or organs receives an equivalent dose in excess of the highest dose in any of the twelve organs for which a weighting factor is specified, a weighting factor of 0.025 should be applied to that tissue or organ and a weighting factor of 0.025 to the average dose in the rest of the remainder as defined above.

cations may be no more than approximations to the true biological situation, but they make it possible to define a radiation field outside the body in dosimetric terms (see Section 2.4) without the need to specify the target organ.

(30) The consequences following an absorbed dose depend not only on the magnitude of the dose, the type and energy of the radiation (dealt with by the radiation weighting factor), and the distribution of the dose within the body (dealt with by the tissue weighting factor), but also on the distribution of the dose in time (dose rate and protraction of exposure). In previous formulations, provision was made for possible weighting factors other than the radiation and tissue weighting factors. The product of these other, unspecified, weighting factors was called N. Any effect of the time distribution of dose could have been accommodated by assigning a set of values to N. In practice this has not been attempted and the Commission has decided to drop the use of N. The effect of all exposure conditions other than those dealt with by the radiation and tissue weighting factors will be covered by using different values of the coefficients relating equivalent dose and effective dose to the probability of stochastic effects, rather than by using additional weighting factors in the definitions of the quantities.

(31) The values of both the radiation and the tissue weighting factors depend on our current knowledge of radiobiology and may change from time to time. Indeed, new values are adopted in these recommendations. Although such changes are infrequent, they can cause confusion. The definitions of equivalent dose (in a single tissue or organ) and effective dose (in the whole body) are not confined to any particular set of values of these weighting factors, so care is needed to avoid ambiguity. When the Commission uses equivalent dose and effective dose, it will be implicit that these contain the values of radiation and tissue weighting factors recommended at the relevant time by the Commission. It is appropriate to treat as additive the weighted quantities used by the Commission but assessed at different times, despite the use of different values of weighting factors. The Commission does not recommend that any attempt be made to correct earlier values. It is also appropriate to add values of dose equivalent to equivalent dose and values of effective dose equivalent to effective dose without any adjustments. If values of weighting factors other than those recommended by the Commission are used, this fact should be clearly stated and the values should be explicitly given when the quantities are introduced. These weighted quantities should not be added to the Commission's quantities.

(32) Both equivalent dose and effective dose are quantities intended for use in radiological protection, including the assessment of risks in general terms. They provide a basis for estimating the probability of stochastic effects only for absorbed doses well below the thresholds for deterministic effects. For the estimation of the likely consequences of an exposure of a known population, it will sometimes be better to use absorbed dose and specific data relating to the relative biological effectiveness of the radiations concerned and the probability coefficients relating to the exposed population.

2.3. Subsidiary Dosimetric Quantities

(33) Several subsidiary dosimetric quantities have proved useful. Following an intake to the body of a radioactive material, there is a period during which the material gives rise to equivalent doses in the tissues of the body at varying rates. The time integral of the equivalent-dose rate is called the **committed equivalent dose**, $H_T(\tau)$ where τ is the integration time (in years) following the intake. If τ is not specified, it is implied that the value is 50 years for adults and from intake to age 70 years for children. By extension, the **committed effective dose**, $E(\tau)$, is similarly defined. When the Commission refers to an equivalent or effective dose accumulated in a given period of time, it is implicit that any committed doses from intakes occurring in that same period are included.

(34) The dosimetric quantities referred to above all relate to the exposure of an individual. The Commission uses further quantities related to exposed groups or populations. These quantities take account of the number of people exposed to a source by multiplying the average dose to the exposed group from the source by the number of individuals in the group. The relevant quantities are the **collective equivalent dose**, S_T, which relates to a specified tissue or organ, and the **collective effective dose**, S. If several groups are involved, the total collective quantity is the sum of the collective quantities for each group. The unit of these collective quantities is the man sievert. The collective quantities can be thought of as representing the total consequences of the exposure of a population or group, but their use in this way should be limited to situations in which the consequences are truly proportional to both the dosimetric quantity and number of people exposed, and in which an appropriate probability coefficient is available (see

Section 2.4). When it is necessary to distinguish between a collective dose and the dose to an individual, the latter is called the individual dose.

(35) The collective effective dose resulting from the presence of radioactive materials in the environment may be accumulated over long periods of time, covering successive generations of individuals. The total collective effective dose to be expected from a given situation is the integral over all time of the collective effective dose rate resulting from, i.e. committed by, a single release (or a unit period of a practice in the case of a continuing operation). If the integration is not over infinite time, the quantity is described as being truncated at a defined time. If the ranges of individual dose or time are large, it may be useful to subdivide the collective quantities into blocks covering more limited ranges of dose and time. When considering the consequences of a unit period of practice, it is sometimes convenient to distinguish between the collective effective dose already delivered and the collective effective dose committed over all time.

(36) **The dose commitment** ($H_{c,T}$ or E_c) is a calculational tool. It can be assessed for a critical group as well as for the whole world population. It is defined as the infinite time integral of the **per caput dose rate** ($\dot{H}_T$ or $\dot{E}$) due to a specified event, such as a unit of practice (e.g. a year of practice):

$$H_{c,T} = \int_0^\infty \dot{H}_T(t) \, dt$$

or

$$E_c = \int_0^\infty \dot{E}(t) \, dt$$

In the case of an indefinite practice at a constant rate, the maximum annual per caput dose rate ($\dot{H}_T$ or $\dot{E}$) in the future for the specified population will be equal to the dose commitment of one year of practice, irrespective of changes in the population size. If the practice is continued only over a time period τ, the maximum future annual per caput dose will be equal to the corresponding truncated dose commitment, defined as

$$H_{c,T}(\tau) = \int_0^\tau \dot{H}_T(t) \, dt$$

or

$$E_c(\tau) = \int_0^\tau \dot{E}(t) \, dt$$

2.4. Other Quantities

(37) Several other quantities are of special use in radiological protection. One of these is the **activity**, A, of a quantity of a radionuclide. Activity is the average number of spontaneous nuclear transformations taking place per unit time. Its unit is the reciprocal second, s^{-1}, given, for this purpose, the special name becquerel (Bq).

(38) There are also four operational quantities of particular interest in the measurement of radiation fields for protection purposes. These ICRU quantities, the **ambient dose equivalent**, $H^*(d)$, the **directional dose equivalent**, $H'(d)$, the **individual dose equivalent, penetrating**, $H_p(d)$, and the **individual dose equivalent, superficial**, $H_s(d)$ are

defined in Annex A. All these quantities are based on the concept of the dose equivalent at a point and not on the concept of equivalent dose (see paragraph 24).

(39) In relating the probability of stochastic effects to dosimetric quantities, it is convenient to use a probability coefficient. For example, the **fatality probability coefficient** is the quotient of probability that an increment of dose will cause death and the magnitude of that increment of dose. The dose in question will usually be an equivalent dose or an effective dose. Such coefficients necessarily relate to a specified population.

(40) It is often useful in general statements to use generic terms that can apply to any of the relevant dosimetric quantities. The Commission uses "dose" as one such term in phrases such as "dose limit". This may be a limit applied to equivalent or effective dose. The choice is usually clear from the context. The Commission also uses the term "exposure" in a generic sense to mean the process of being exposed to radiation or radioactive material. The significance of an exposure in this sense is determined by the resulting doses. It seems unlikely that this causes any confusion with the highly specific use of exposure as a quantity defined by ICRU.

(41) The Commission uses the International System of units (SI) and the international convention that the names of units are written with a lower case initial letter. The abbreviations for units are written with a lower case letter, or initial letter, except when the name of the unit is derived from a person's name, e.g. m and mm for metre and millimetre, but Sv and mSv for sievert and millisievert.

3. BIOLOGICAL ASPECTS OF RADIOLOGICAL PROTECTION

Chapter 3 provides an introduction to the stochastic and deterministic biological effects of ionising radiation and leads on to a discussion of the problems of establishing a quantitative measure of the detriment associated with an exposure to radiation. More detailed biological information, including that on radiation risks, is provided in Annex B. The use of this information as a basis for radiological protection policy is discussed in Annex C.

3.1. Introduction

(42) As explained in Chapter 1, radiological protection is concerned with protecting man against the harmful effects of radiation. In all its work, the Commission has based its approach on the best available information on the biological effects of radiation and has used this to provide a simplified, but adequate, biological basis for radiological protection. This chapter and Annex B therefore deal with the deleterious effects only to the extent necessary to support that approach. To help in achieving clarity, distinction has been made between four terms: change, damage, harm and detriment. Changes may or may not be harmful. Damage represents some degree of deleterious change, for example to cells, but is not necessarily deleterious to the exposed individual. Harm is the term used to denote clinically observable deleterious effects that are expressed in individuals (somatic effects) or their descendants (hereditary effects). Detriment is a complex concept combining the probability, severity and time of expression of harm. It is not easily represented by a single variable and is discussed in Section 3.3.

(43) The term "risk" has previously been used by the Commission to mean the probability of a defined deleterious outcome, but it has also been widely used elsewhere

as the product of the probability and severity of an event and, more generally, in a purely descriptive manner. The Commission now uses risk only descriptively and in well-established expressions such as "risk estimate" and "excess relative risk". It now uses probability when that is what is meant. Aspects of probability and risk are discussed in detail in Annexes B and C.

3.2. The Biological Effects of Ionising Radiation

(44) Part of this material has been previewed in Section 2.1, and is discussed here in more detail. The process of ionisation necessarily changes atoms, at least transiently, and may thus alter the structure of the molecules containing them. Molecular changes may also be caused by the excitation of atoms and molecules if the excitation energy exceeds the binding energy between atoms. About half the energy deposited in tissue by ionising radiation is due to excitation, but this is of less consequence than ionisation and has not been considered separately in what follows. If the affected molecules are in a living cell, the cell itself may sometimes be damaged, either directly if the molecule is critical to the cell's function, or indirectly by causing chemical changes in adjacent molecules, e.g. the production of free radicals. Of the various forms of damage that radiation can cause in cells, the most important is that in the DNA. Damage in the DNA may prevent the survival or reproduction of the cell, but frequently the damage is repaired by the cell. If that repair is not perfect, it may result in a viable but modified cell. The occurrence and proliferation of a modified cell may well be influenced by other changes in the cell caused either before or after the exposure to radiation. Such influences are common and may include exposure to other carcinogens or mutagens.

(45) If enough cells in an organ or tissue are killed or prevented from reproducing and functioning normally, there will be a loss of organ function—an effect that the Commission now calls "deterministic". The loss of function will become more serious as the number of affected cells is increased. More details are given in Section 3.4.1. A modified somatic cell may still retain its reproductive capacity and may give rise to a clone of modified cells that may eventually result in a cancer. A modified germ cell in the gonads, with the function of transmitting genetic information to the descendants of an exposed individual, may transmit incorrect hereditary information and may cause severe harm to some of those descendants. These somatic and hereditary effects, which may start from a single modified cell, are called stochastic effects. They are discussed further in Sections 3.4.2 and 3.4.3. Because of the complex processes involved in the development of the conceptus to an embryo and a fetus, it is convenient to discuss both deterministic and stochastic effects of radiation on the unborn child in a separate section (Section 3.4.4).

(46) There is some experimental evidence that radiation can act to stimulate a variety of cellular functions, including proliferation and repair. Such stimulation is not necessarily beneficial. In some circumstances, radiation appears also to enhance immunological responses and to modify the balance of hormones in the body. In particular, radiation may be able to stimulate the repair of prior radiation damage, thus decreasing its consequences, or may be able to improve immunological surveillance, thus strengthening the body's natural defence mechanisms. Most of the experimental data on such effects, currently termed "hormesis", have been inconclusive, mainly because of statistical difficulties at low doses. Furthermore, many relate to biological endpoints other than cancer or hereditary effects. The available data on hormesis are not sufficient to take them into account in radiological protection.

3.3. The Concept of Detriment

(47) In *Publication 26* (1977), the Commission introduced the concept of **detriment** as a measure of the total harm that would eventually be experienced by an exposed group and its descendants as a result of the group's exposure to a radiation source. Health detriment was included as part of the total detriment. In practice, the Commission has used only the health detriment and recommends that a separate allowance should be made for other forms of detriment when decision-aiding techniques are used, for example in optimisation studies. In this report, the Commission uses the term detriment to mean only health detriment.

(48) The Commission's definition of detriment in *Publication 26* used the expected number of cases of a radiation-induced health effect weighted by a factor representing the severity of the effect. It was the expectation value (called more strictly the mathematical expectation) of the weighted number of health effects to be experienced by the group. The weighting factor was taken as 1 for the death of individuals and for severe hereditary effects in their descendants. Smaller weighting factors were implied for other, less severe effects, but were not specified. In relation to an individual, the detriment could also be expressed as the product of the probability of a deleterious effect and a measure of the severity of that effect. If the measure of the severity is normalised to 1 for the most severe effects, and if the values of all the products are small, the products for different outcomes in the same individual can be summed to give the total detriment to that individual. It is implicit in this concept of detriment that the relevant doses are small, well below the thresholds for deterministic effects.

(49) This approach to detriment has proved useful but is somewhat too limited. The Commission now finds it necessary to take a broader view. The general aim is still to find a quantitative way of expressing a combination of the probability of occurrence of a health effect and a judgement of the severity of that effect. Ideally, detriment should be represented as an extensive quantity, i.e. one that allows the detriment to a group to be added as additional exposures occur to individuals and as more individuals are added to the group. This requirement cannot be fully met, at least for the individual, because some of the outcomes of exposure are mutually exclusive and some are not. Death due to one exposure excludes death due to another, but non-fatal conditions may occur concurrently or consecutively. A second problem is posed by the multifarious nature of the possible outcomes, so that probability and severity can be combined in many different ways to represent detriment.

(50) The Commission needs to use detriment for several different purposes. One is to assess the consequences of continued or cumulative exposures in order to recommend dose limits. Another is to compare the consequences of different distributions of equivalent dose within the body and thence to select a set of tissue weighting factors. A third is to provide a basis for assessing the valuation of a unit of effective dose for use, for example, in the optimisation of protection within a practice. These purposes are discussed in Chapter 4.

(51) The Commission has concluded that the many aspects of detriment and its many purposes make the selection of a single approach undesirable. Therefore, the Commission has replaced its previous concept of detriment by a multi-dimensional concept. For recommending dose limits, the detriment from an exposure has been expressed in a variety of ways. This approach is dealt with in Chapter 5 and, in more detail, in Annexes B and C. For this purpose, only a limited attempt is made to aggregate these facets into a

single quantity, called in *Publication 45* (1985) a unified index of harm. However, an aggregative method was preferred in choosing tissue weighting factors because these are used only to make adjustments for the differential sensitivity of tissues and organs. Since it is rare for single tissues, except for the lung and perhaps the thyroid and skin, to be irradiated alone, the choice of tissue weighting factors is not very sensitive to the procedure for aggregating the different aspects of detriment. Details are given in Section 3.5 and in Annex B.

3.4. Quantitative Estimates of the Consequences of Radiation Exposures

(52) In order to develop a system of radiological protection, it is necessary to know quantitatively how the probability of stochastic effects and the severity of deterministic effects vary with dose. The most relevant sources of information are those obtained directly from studies of the effects of radiation on man. In addition, a great deal of information about the mechanisms of damage and the relationships between dose and the probability of deleterious effects in man can be inferred from studies on micro-organisms, on isolated cells grown *in vitro*, and on animals. Unfortunately, little, if any, of the available information can be applied directly in radiological protection—it all needs considerable interpretation. The Commission's conclusions on the biological information needed in radiological protection are drawn to the maximum extent possible from data on radiation effects in human beings, with other information used in support.

(53) Data on deterministic effects in man come from the side effects of radiotherapy, from effects on the early radiologists, from the effects of the atomic bombs at Hiroshima and Nagasaki in Japan, and from the consequences of severe accidents, some in the nuclear industry and some involving radiographic sources. At present, the three principal sources of information on stochastic effects are the epidemiological studies on the survivors of the nuclear weapon attacks on Hiroshima and Nagasaki, on patients exposed to radiation for medical treatment or diagnosis, and on some groups of workers exposed to radiation or radioactive substances at work. Studies of this kind are very complex and time-consuming and are not conducted by the Commission itself. The Commission, with the help of its Committees, examines the published accounts of the studies and any reviews carried out by national and international bodies and then draws conclusions relevant to the needs of radiological protection.

3.4.1. *Deterministic effects*

(54) In many organs and tissues of the body there is a continuous process of loss and replacement of cells. An increase in the rate of loss, for example following exposure to radiation, may be compensated for by an increase in the replacement rate, but there will be a transient, and sometimes permanent, net reduction in the number of cells available to maintain the functions of the organ or tissue. Many organs and tissues are unaffected by small reductions in the number of available cells, but if the decrease is large enough, there will be clinically observable pathological conditions such as a loss of tissue function or a consequential reaction as the body attempts to repair the damage. If the tissue is vital and is damaged sufficiently, the end result will be death. If some individuals in the exposed group are already in a state of health approaching the pathological condition, they will reach that condition as a result of exposure to radiation after a smaller loss of cells than would usually be the case. For healthy individuals, the probability of causing harm will be zero at doses up to some hundreds, or sometimes thousands, of milli-

sieverts, depending on the tissue, and will increase steeply to unity (100%) above some level of dose called the threshold, more strictly, the threshold for clinical effect. The plot on linear axes of the probability of harm against dose is sigmoid. Above the appropriate threshold, the severity of the harm will increase with dose, reflecting the number of cells damaged, and usually with dose rate because a protracted dose will cause the damage to cells to be spread out in time, allowing for more effective repair or repopulation. This type of effect, characterised by a severity that increases with dose above some clinical threshold, was previously called "non-stochastic". Although the initial cellular changes are essentially random, the large number of cells involved in the initiation of a clinically observable, non-stochastic effect gives the effect a deterministic character. For this reason, the Commission now calls such effects "deterministic" effects.

(55) In addition to the loss of functional cells in a tissue or organ, damage to supporting blood vessels may also occur, leading to secondary tissue damage. There may also be some replacement of functional cells by fibrous tissue causing a reduction in organ function. The clinical findings depend on the specific function of the irradiated tissue. For example, opacities may occur in the lens of the eye, sometimes leading to visual impairment (cataract), and, if the gonads are irradiated, there may be a temporary or permanent loss of fertility.

(56) Some deterministic effects are of a functional nature and may be reversible, provided that the damage is not too severe. Some examples of functional effects are: decreasing of glandular secretions (e.g. from the salivary glands or thyroid); neurological effects (e.g. changes in electroencephalograms or retinograms); vascular reactions (e.g. early erythema or subcutaneous oedema).

(57) The equivalent dose is not always the appropriate quantity for use in relation to deterministic effects because the values of radiation weighting factors have been chosen to reflect the relative biological effectiveness (RBE) of the different types and energies of radiation in producing stochastic effects. For radiations with a radiation weighting factor larger than 1, the values of RBE for deterministic effects are smaller than those for stochastic effects. The use of the equivalent dose to predict deterministic effects for high LET radiations, e.g. neutrons, will thus lead to overestimates.

(58) The data for low LET radiation show a wide range of sensitivities for different tissues. However, it can be concluded that few tissues show clinically significant detrimental effects following single (i.e. acute) absorbed doses of less than a few gray. For doses spread out over a period of years, severe effects are not likely in most tissues at annual doses of less than about 0.5 Gy. However, the gonads, the lens of the eye, and the bone marrow show higher sensitivities.

(59) The threshold for temporary sterility in the male for a single absorbed dose in the testes is about 0.15 Gy. Under conditions of prolonged exposure the dose rate threshold is about 0.4 Gy y^{-1}. The corresponding values for permanent sterility are about 3.5 to 6 Gy and 2 Gy y^{-1}. The threshold for permanent sterility in women is an acute absorbed dose in the range from about 2.5 to 6 Gy, older women being more sensitive; or a protracted dose rate over many years of more than 0.2 Gy y^{-1} (see Annex B, Table B-1).

(60) The threshold for opacities sufficient to cause impairment of vision, which occur after some delay, seems to be in the range 2 to 10 Gy for an acute exposure to low LET radiation. For high LET radiation, the absorbed dose thresholds are 2 or 3 times less. The dose rate threshold is less well known for chronic exposure, but for exposure over many years is thought to be somewhat above 0.15 Gy y^{-1} (see Annex B, Table B-1).

(61) Clinically significant depression of the blood-forming process has a threshold for

acute absorbed doses in the whole bone marrow of about 0.5 Gy. The dose-rate threshold for protracted exposure over many years is more than 0.4 Gy y^{-1}. The LD_{50} in 60 days due to bone marrow syndrome in a heterogeneous population uniformly and acutely exposed is about 3 to 5 Gy in the absence of a high standard of medical care (see Annex B, Table B-2).

3.4.2. *Stochastic effects in exposed individuals*

(62) The response of the body to the development of a clone of modified somatic cells is complex. The initial development of such a clone may be inhibited unless its development is promoted by some additional agent and any surviving clone is very likely to be eliminated or isolated by the body's defences. However, if it is not, it may result, after a prolonged and variable delay called the latency period, in the development of a malignant condition in which the proliferation of modified cells is uncontrolled. Such conditions are commonly grouped together and called cancer. The cancers induced by radiation, with or without a contribution from other agents, are not distinguishable from those occurring from other causes. The defence mechanisms are not likely to be totally effective, even at small doses, so they are unlikely to give rise to a threshold in the dose–response relationship. The probability of a cancer resulting from the radiation will be at least partly dependent on the number of clones of modified cells initially created, since this number will influence the probability of at least one clone surviving. It is then the probability of malignancy that is related to dose, while the severity of a particular cancer is influenced only by the type and location of the malignant condition. The process appears to be random, although individuals may differ somewhat in their sensitivities to the induction of cancer by radiation, reflecting genetic and physiological variations. Some individuals with rare genetic diseases may be substantially more sensitive than the mean. It seems that no stochastic effects in the exposed individual other than cancer (and benign tumours in some organs) are induced by radiation. In particular, any life-shortening found in exposed human populations and in experimental animals after low doses has been shown to be due to excess radiation-induced cancer mortality.

(63) Many million million ion pairs are created every year in the total mass of DNA in a human being by the exposure of the body to natural sources of radiation. No more than about one death in four is attributable to cancer and radiation is responsible for only a small fraction of these cancer deaths. Clearly, the process of passing from the creation of an ion pair in the DNA to the manifestation of a cancer is very rarely completed.

(64) The process of drawing conclusions about stochastic effects is not straightforward because epidemiological studies cannot provide exactly the information needed. They can provide only statistical associations, but they are strengthened when the association is clearly dose-related and is supported by corresponding experimental data. The data from Japan are compelling and are extensive, but they relate to a study group of which about 60% now survive, so the total number of stochastic effects eventually occurring has to be estimated. Moreover, most of the cancers yet to appear will occur in individuals who were under the age of 20 years at the time of exposure, and for whom the attributable lifetime fatality probability per unit dose is probably higher than that for older individuals. Although the study group is large (about 80,000), excess numbers of malignancies, statistically significant at the 95% level, can be found only at doses exceeding about 0.2 Sv. Excesses of lower significance can be found at doses in the region of 0.05 Sv. It must also be borne in mind that all the doses to the Japanese study group were incurred at very high dose rates, whereas information is needed in radiological protection for both acute and protracted exposures, almost always at very much

lower dose rates. However, studies on this group have several advantages over other studies. The group contains both sexes and all ages, and was exposed to a very wide range of doses, from trivial to fatal, distributed fairly uniformly through the bodies of those exposed.

(65) The studies on patients also pose problems. In particular, the irradiations were intentionally non-uniform, the selection of patients on medical grounds sometimes makes it difficult to identify comparable control groups, and the patients may not be representative of the general population. Nevertheless, such groups provide valuable sources of information and are the subject of continuing study.

(66) The studies on workers that have so far yielded significant results relate to those who worked with radium-226 in the early decades of the 20th century and to those who inhaled radon and its daughters in mining, mainly uranium mining, in the middle years of the century. In both cases, there were difficulties in estimating the intake of radioactive materials and the uranium miners may also have been exposed to other carcinogens. The exposures were protracted, but the doses were to localised tissues in the bone and lung and were essentially confined to those from alpha particles. Comparison with the effects of gamma radiation is not simple. Studies on the early radiologists show some stochastic effects, but the estimation of dose is not easy, and quantitative risk estimates have not proved possible. Studies on other groups of workers, such as those in atomic energy laboratories in the US and the UK have provided estimates of risk, with however, very wide confidence intervals. Their range of estimates includes the nominal fatal probability coefficients given in this report.

(67) Numerous reports involving the exposure of populations to low doses of radiation appear in the literature from time to time and are carefully examined by the Commission. Some of these arise from exposure to nuclear sources such as fallout, some involve military personnel exposed at weapons tests and some in the environment of nuclear plants. Others include fetuses exposed to diagnostic x rays, other medically irradiated populations and still other populations living in relatively high natural radiation background areas in the world, including those in India, Brazil, Colorado USA and China. Such low-dose studies avoid the need for the application of factors from high dose-rate information to low dose-rate circumstances, i.e. the DDREF (see paragraph 74). On the other hand, these studies suffer from one or more of the following methodological difficulties including small sample size, lack of adequate controls, extraneous effects other than those due to radiation, inadequate dosimetry and confounding social factors. Furthermore "positive" findings tend to be reported while negative studies often are not. Overall, studies at low dose, while potentially highly relevant to the radiation protection problem, have contributed little to quantitative estimates of risk.

(68) If, as seems likely, some types of cancer can result from the damage originating in a single cell, there can be a real threshold in the dose–response relationship for those types of cancer only if the defence mechanisms are totally successful at small doses. The balance of damage and repair in the cell and the existence of subsequent defence mechanisms can influence the shape of the relationship, but they cannot be expected to result in a real threshold.

(69) At small increments of dose above background, the probability of inducing an additional cancer is certainly small and the expectation value of the number of cases attributable to the increment of dose in an exposed group may well be much less than 1, even in a large group. It is then almost certain that there will be no additional cases, but this provides no evidence for the existence of a real threshold.

(70) In almost all situations apart from accidents and the treatment of patients, the

equivalent dose in individuals is incurred over long periods of time and at annual rates that do not add greatly to the dose delivered to the whole body by natural sources. The annual addition from artificial sources ranges typically from a small fraction of the annual dose from natural sources up to about ten times that annual dose. The lung is a special case because the equivalent dose from radon daughters is very variable and is sometimes as much as several thousand times higher than the equivalent dose to other parts of the body from natural sources.

(71) The existence of doses in all parts of the body from natural sources of radiation decreases the importance of the shape of the dose–response relationship at doses close to zero. Small doses are always additions to the natural background dose. For moderate increments above the background, a linear relationship between the incremental dose and the incremental probability of a deleterious effect will be an adequate approximation, whatever may be the true shape of the relationship between equivalent dose and the probability of stochastic effects. Even so, the shape of this relationship is still important because it can change the estimates of the slope of the incremental relationship.

(72) The simplest relationship between an increment in equivalent dose and the resulting increment in the probability of a defined stochastic effect is that of a straight line through the origin. The human epidemiological data are not sufficiently precise to confirm or exclude that relationship. However, almost all the data relating to stochastic changes in cells *in vitro* and in simple biological organisms such as tradescantia, and to the induction of many animal tumours, show curvilinear dose–effect relationships for radiations of low linear energy transfer (LET), with the slope at low doses being less than that at high doses. In this context, low doses (and low dose rates) imply situations in which it is very unlikely that more than one ionising event will occur in the critical parts of a cell within the time during which repair mechanisms in the cell can operate. In such situations, the dose–response relationship will be linear. At higher doses and dose rates, two or more events may be able to combine, producing an enhanced effect reflected by a quadratic term in the dose–response relationship. At still higher doses, where cell killing becomes important, the slope again decreases. The results for radiations of high LET are usually more nearly rectilinear over the range of doses below those causing appreciable cell killing. Some cellular studies *in vitro*, however, show an increased slope at the low-dose end of this range.

(73) In short, for low LET radiations, the most characteristic form of the relationship between the equivalent dose in an organ and the probability of a resultant cancer is that of an initial proportional response at low values of equivalent dose, followed by a steeper rate of increase (slope) that can be represented by a quadratic term, followed finally by a decreasing slope due to cell killing. There are no adequate grounds for assuming a real threshold in the relationship. This form of response, while typical, is not necessarily the definitive form for all human cancers. Taken together with the linear approximation for increments over the dose due to natural background, it provides a suitable basis for the Commission's use of a simple proportional relationship at all levels of equivalent dose and effective dose below the dose limits recommended in this report.

(74) The Commission has concluded that, in the context of radiological protection, there is sufficient evidence to justify its making an allowance for non-linearity when interpreting data for low LET radiation at high doses and high dose rates to give estimates of the probability of effects at low doses and low dose rates. On the basis of discussions in Annex B, the Commission has decided to reduce by a factor of 2 the probability co-

efficients obtained directly from observations at high doses and high dose rates, modified if necessary by an allowance for the effects of cell killing. There is a wide spread in the data and the Commission recognises that the choice of this value is somewhat arbitrary and may be conservative. No such factor is used in the interpretation of data for high LET radiation. The reduction factor is called by the Commission the **Dose and Dose Rate Effectiveness Factor**, DDREF. It has been included in the probability coefficients for all equivalent doses resulting from absorbed doses below 0.2 Gy and from higher absorbed doses when the dose rate is less than 0.1 Gy per hour.

(75) Another major difficulty in interpreting the human data is that of estimating the number of stochastic effects yet to appear in the populations being studied. For a few cancers, there is no difficulty because the rate of appearance of new cases has fallen back to, or close to, the expected rate in a matched control population. This is true of leukaemia in the Japanese survivors and the British spondylitics and of bone cancer in the patients injected with radium-224. For the total of other cancers, the rate is still enhanced and, in the Japanese study, still rising, largely as a result of the excess mortality in those exposed as children.

(76) For most types of cancer, the excess mortality seems, after an initial period of zero or very low risk called the minimum latency period, to have the same pattern in time as the natural mortality due to the same type of cancer. If this pattern is continued throughout life, and this is by no means certain, there will be a simple proportion between the natural cancer mortality and the excess due to radiation for the whole time after the minimum latency period. This model, the **multiplicative risk projection model**, is probably too simple, even for the exposure of adults. The Japanese data show that neither it nor the additive risk projection model (see below) adequately fits the pattern of mortality following the exposure of young children. The model does not necessarily imply a multiplicative biological process—it may only be a convenient description of the way in which the probability of an attributable cancer varies with time after exposure.

(77) An alternative model, the **additive risk projection model**, postulates that the excess mortality would be broadly independent of the natural mortality. After the initial minimum latency period, the rate would rise over a period of years after exposure and then remain fairly constant or, as with leukaemia and bone cancer, fall. This model, with current probability coefficients, produces predictions of eventual total probability of death of about half the values predicted by the multiplicative risk projection. It also predicts more time lost per attributable death. However, it is no longer seen to be consistent with most of the epidemiological observations.

(78) Because of the uncertainties of recording cancer incidence rather than mortality, most of the data on exposed human populations are expressed in terms of excess cancer mortality attributable to the exposures. However, the incidence of cancer is also important and the Commission takes it into account on the basis of currently observed cure rate for the main types of cancer. More generally, the Commission needs a broader basis for expressing the harm expected in an exposed population and has therefore made use of the concept of detriment as discussed in Section 3.3. Hereditary effects are discussed in Section 3.4.3.

(79) All these difficulties introduce uncertainties into the estimation of the cancer risks from exposure to radiation. For this reason, and because the Commission estimates the risks for representative populations with defined exposure patterns, the Commission calls the estimated probability of a fatal cancer per unit effective dose the **nominal fatality probability coefficient**. This applies to low doses at all dose rates and to high doses and

low dose rates (see paragraph 74). In deriving values of the nominal probability co-efficient, the Commission has previously used the probability of induction of a fatal cancer without making any allowance for the reduction in that probability resulting from competing causes of death. If a multiplicative, rather than additive, risk projection model is used, that correction is essential. The correction is now used by the Commission in deriving all values of probability coefficients. As will be discussed in Chapter 5, it is very desirable for protection purposes to use the same nominal coefficients for both men and women and for a representative population of a wide range of ages. Although there are differences between the sexes and between populations of different age-specific mortality rates, these are not so large as to necessitate the use by the Commission of different nominal probability coefficients. A small difference is, however, introduced between the nominal probability coefficients for workers and for the whole population. Although small, this difference is very likely to exist because it arises principally from the inclusion of the more sensitive younger age groups in the whole population.

(80) Reviews of the available data are summarised in Annex B. In choosing a value for the nominal probability coefficients, the Commission has had to take account of a wide range of options. Because the data from Japan are derived from a large population of all ages and both sexes, and because the doses are fairly uniformly distributed through the whole body, these data have been taken as the primary source of information. The interpretation of the data from the irradiated spondylitic patients leads to a lower estimate of the annual probability of fatal cancer per unit dose by a factor of about two. Lower estimates can also be derived from studies on patients treated for cervical cancer, although the doses were very non-uniform. These data confirm the Commission's view that the estimates based on the data from Hiroshima and Nagasaki are unlikely to underestimate the risks.

(81) The Commission has also had to select a risk projection model. For leukaemia, the choice of model has little effect because it is likely that almost all the leukaemia deaths have already been observed. The combination of models used by the Commission emphasises the multiplicative model for cancers other than leukaemia, with the understanding that this may overestimate the probability of cancer incidence at older ages because the multiplying factor may not persist over the whole span of life. The effect of competing causes of death reduces the importance of any such error.

(82) Finally, the Commission has had to decide how to transfer conclusions reached about the post-war Japanese population to other populations. Again two models are available. Either the absolute mortality rate per unit dose can be applied to the other populations or the transfer can be made by using the proportional increase in the mortality rate of each type of cancer in turn. In either case, the mortality pattern of the new population has to be used to allow for competing causes of death. The Commission has averaged over five populations to give a reasonable representation of a typical population. There is no adequate basis at present for making a choice between the two transfer models and the Commission has used the average of both methods.

(83) The data in Annex B relating to high doses and high dose rates of low LET radiation, show a lifetime fatality probability coefficient for a reference population of both sexes and of working age, of about 8×10^{-2} Sv^{-1} for the sum of all malignancies. This value, combined with the DDREF of 2, leads to a nominal probability coefficient for workers of 4×10^{-2} Sv^{-1}. The corresponding values for the whole population, including children, are about 10×10^{-2} Sv^{-1} for high doses and dose rates and 5×10^{-2} Sv^{-1} for low dose and dose rates (see Table 3). Typically, the multiplicative model shows a mean

loss of life per attributable cancer death of about 13 to 15 years. The additive model gives a corresponding figure of about 20 years.

(84) Extensive data exist on the relationship between the probability of bone cancer and the radium content of workers in the early luminising industry; between the probability of bone cancer in patients and the activity of radium-224 injected; and between the probability of lung cancer and the estimated exposure to radon and its daughters in mining environments. In almost all these cases, it is difficult to estimate the dosimetric quantities and thus these human data do not provide good estimates of the relationship between the stochastic effects from exposure to high LET radiation and the doses to human organs. However, it is known from studies on cells and from work with experimental animals that, per unit absorbed dose, high LET radiations cause more stochastic damage than do low LET radiations.

(85) Values of the relative biological effectiveness do not lead directly to values of the radiation weighting factor. Experimental data from animals and cells are used to estimate the relevant values of RBE for typical stochastic effects at low doses. The experimental studies use either x rays with an energy of a few hundred keV or gamma rays of energy of about 1 MeV. While these radiations are about equally effective at high doses and high dose rates, there is a factor of about two in biological effectiveness between these two energy bands at low doses. Since the values of radiation weighting factor have to apply to all the tissues and organs in the body, a substantial degree of simplification is needed. The Commission has therefore not distinguished between x and gamma radiation and has selected values of radiation weighting factor for other radiations broadly representative of the observed values of RBE relative to either x or gamma radiation. The nominal fatality probability coefficients per unit equivalent dose and per unit effective dose for high LET radiation are then the same as those for low LET radiation. The values are given in Table 1 in Chapter 2.

(86) In the special case of lung cancer from inhaled radon progeny, the epidemiological data from radon-exposed miners yield a direct relationship between their cumulative exposure to radon progeny and the excess probability of lung cancer (see Annex B). In these circumstances it is reasonable to express the attributable risk coefficient per unit of radon exposure and not per unit dose to the lung or the bronchial epithelium.

3.4.3. *Stochastic effects in progeny*

(87) If the damage caused by radiation occurs in the germ cells, this damage (mutations and chromosomal aberrations) may be transmitted and become manifest as hereditary disorders in the descendants of the exposed individual. Radiation has not been identified as a cause of such effects in man, but experimental studies on plants and animals suggest that such effects will occur and that the consequences may range from the undetectably trivial, through gross malformations or loss of function, to premature death. It must be presumed that any non-lethal damage in human germ cells may be further transmitted to subsequent generations. This type of stochastic effect is called "hereditary".

(88) Hereditary effects vary widely in their severity. One such effect is the production of dominant mutations leading to genetic disease in the first generation progeny. Some of these conditions are seriously harmful to the affected individual and are sometimes life-threatening. They occur predominantly in the first and second generations after exposure. Chromosomal aberrations may also result in congenital abnormalities in children.

Recessive mutations produce little effect in the first few generations of descendants, but make a contribution to the general pool of genetic damage in subsequent generations. There are also many deleterious conditions that have a substantial incidence in man and which are due to the interaction of genetic and environmental factors. They are known as multifactorial disorders. A general increase in mutations might increase their incidence, although this has not been demonstrated in either man or animals. In assessing the consequences for exposed individuals, the Commission has previously taken account of the hereditary effects that might occur in their children and grandchildren. This left the effects in later generations to be considered as part of the consequences for society. The Commission now attributes the whole detriment to the dose received by the exposed individual, thus avoiding the need for a two-stage assessment.

(89) For low doses and dose rates, the nominal hereditary effect probability coefficient for severe effects (excluding multifactorial effects, see below) over all generations and related to the gonad doses distributed over the whole population is 0.5×10^{-2} Sv^{-1}. About 80% of the effects are due to dominant and X-linked mutations. Of these, about 15% occur in each of the first two generations. No reliable estimate is available for the probability coefficient for the multifactorial conditions, but, weighted for severity, it is probably about 0.5×10^{-2} Sv^{-1}. Because of the different age distribution of a working population, the coefficients for workers are slightly smaller than for the general population (a reduction by about 40%). The Commission considers that the nominal hereditary effect probability coefficients of 1×10^{-2} Sv^{-1} for the whole population and 0.6×10^{-2} Sv^{-1} for workers adequately represent the weighted number of hereditary effects to be expected in all generations (see Table 3). This only includes weighting for severity. With further weighting for years of life lost if the harm occurs (see paragraph 96), the corresponding numbers will be 1.3×10^{-2} Sv^{-1} and 0.8×10^{-2} Sv^{-1} (see Table 4).

Table 3. Nominal probability coefficients for stochastic effects

| Exposed population | Detriment $(10^{-2}$ $Sv^{-1})$[1] | | | |
	Fatal cancer[2]	Non-fatal cancer	Severe hereditary effects	Total
Adult workers	4.0	0.8	0.8	5.6
Whole population	5.0	1.0	1.3	7.3

[1] Rounded values.
[2] For fatal cancer, the detriment coefficient is equal to the probability coefficient.

3.4.4. *Effects of antenatal exposure*

(90) The effects on the conceptus of exposure to radiation depend on the time of exposure relative to conception. When the number of cells in the conceptus is small and their nature is not yet specialised, the effect of damage to these cells is most likely to take the form of a failure to implant or of an undetectable death of the conceptus. It is thought that any cellular damage at this stage is much more likely to cause the death of the conceptus than to result in stochastic effects expressed in the live-born. Exposure of the embryo in the first three weeks following conception is not likely to result in deterministic or stochastic effects in the live-born child, despite the fact that the central nervous system and the heart are beginning to develop in the third week. During the rest

of the period of major organogenesis, conventionally taken to be from the start of the third week after conception, malformations may be caused in the organ under development at time of exposure. These effects are deterministic in character with a threshold in man, estimated from animal experiments, to be about 0.1 Gy.

(91) Throughout the period from 3 weeks after conception until the end of pregnancy, it is likely that radiation exposure can cause stochastic effects resulting in an increased probability of cancer in the live-born. The available data are not consistent and considerable uncertainty exists. However, the Commission assumes that the nominal fatality probability coefficient is, at most, a few times that for the population as a whole.

(92) Values of intelligence quotient (IQ) lower than expected have been reported in some children exposed in utero at Hiroshima and Nagasaki. There have been two principal quantitative findings. One is the observation of a general downward shift in the distribution of IQ with increasing dose. The Commission assumes that the shift is proportional to dose. Small shifts cannot be clinically identified. A coefficient of about 30 IQ points Sv^{-1} relates to the dose in the fetus in the period from 8 weeks to 15 weeks after conception. A similar, but smaller shift, is detectable following exposure in the period from 16 weeks to 25 weeks. This appears to be a deterministic effect, probably with a threshold determined only by the minimum shift in IQ that can be clinically recognised.

(93) The second finding is of a dose-related increase in the frequency of children classified as "severely retarded". The number of cases is small, but the data indicate an excess probability of severe mental retardation of 0.4 at 1 Sv. As shown in Annex B, this finding is consistent with the general shift in IQ distribution with increasing dose. Because of the Gaussian shape of the IQ distribution, the excess number of cases of severe mental retardation will be very small at small IQ shifts, rising steeply only as the shift approaches 30 IQ points. On this basis, a large change in the IQ of an individual can be caused only by a large dose. At doses of the order of 0.1 Sv, no effect would be detectable in the general distribution of IQ, but at somewhat larger doses the effect might be sufficient to show an increase in the number of children classified as severely retarded. The effects at all levels of dose are less marked following exposure in the period from 16 weeks to 25 weeks after conception and have not been observed for other periods. All the observations on IQ and severe mental retardation relate to high dose and high-dose rates and their direct use probably overestimates the risks.

3.5. Tissue Weighting Factors

(94) The tissue weighting factors introduced in Chapter 2 for defining the quantity effective dose were intended to ensure that a weighted tissue equivalent dose would produce broadly the same degree of detriment irrespective of the tissue or organ involved. The Commission has adopted an aggregated representation of detriment for this purpose. It includes four components: the probability of attributable fatal cancer, the weighted probability of attributable non-fatal cancer, the weighted probability of severe hereditary effects and the relative length of life lost. Since effective dose will be used only over ranges where the total probability of attributable death will be small, even the fatal contribution to detriment can be treated as additive when several organs are irradiated. Each consequence can then be weighted by a factor chosen to represent its severity. As in *Publication 26*, death and severe hereditary effects are both given a weighting factor of 1.

(95) Discussions in *Publication 45* (1985) suggest a weight for non-fatal cancers relative to fatal cancers equal to the average lethality fraction of the cancer concerned. A type of cancer that is difficult to cure, and thus has a high lethality fraction and usually a reduced quality of life for the survivors, would have a high weighting factor for the non-fatal events, while an easily cured cancer would have a low weighting factor for the non-fatal events. The weights would then range from about 0.01 for non-fatal skin cancer to about 0.99 for non-fatal leukaemia. The weighting factor to be applied to the fatality coefficient is derived in Annex B. The weighting factors for the severity of hereditary effects is already included in the probability coefficients.

(96) A second weighting is applied to take account of the different mean latency time for different types of cancer. This weighting is simply the relative time lost due to an attributable cancer death or, in the case of non-fatal cancers and hereditary effects, the relative time of impaired life taken for cancers as the same as the time lost by death for the same type of cancer. Finally, the products of the mortality coefficient and the weighting factors for morbidity and time lost are normalised to give a total of unity and thus provide a basis for the tissue weighting factors recommended by the Commission. These tissue weighting factors are provided as rounded values for individual tissues and organs and are given in Table 2 on bases set out in Annex B.

(97) The data in Table 4 are representative of those for a nominal population of equal numbers of men and women. Except for the breast, the differences between the sexes are small. The effect on the tissue weighting factors of combining the data is that some weighting factors are slightly higher and some slightly lower than the values that would relate to men and women separately. The effect of confining the population to workers is

Table 4. Nominal probability coefficients for individual tissues and organs[1]

Tissue or organ	Probability of fatal cancer $(10^{-2}\ Sv^{-1})$		Aggregated detriment[2] $(10^{-2}\ Sv^{-1})$	
	Whole population	Workers	Whole population	Workers
Bladder	0.30	0.24	0.29	0.24
Bone marrow	0.50	0.40	1.04	0.83
Bone surface	0.05	0.04	0.07	0.06
Breast	0.20	0.16	0.36	0.29
Colon	0.85	0.68	1.03	0.82
Liver	0.15	0.12	0.16	0.13
Lung	0.85	0.68	0.80	0.64
Oesophagus	0.30	0.24	0.24	0.19
Ovary	0.10	0.08	0.15	0.12
Skin	0.02	0.02	0.04	0.03
Stomach	1.10	0.88	1.00	0.80
Thyroid	0.08	0.06	0.15	0.12
Remainder	0.50	0.40	0.59	0.47
Total	5.00	4.00	5.92	4.74
	Probability of severe hereditary disorders			
Gonads	1.00	0.6	1.33	0.80
Grand total (rounded)			7.3	5.6

[1] The values relate to a population of equal numbers of both sexes and a wide range of ages.
[2] See paragraphs 95 and 96 and Table B-20 in Annex B.

to decrease the nominal probability coefficient for workers to 4×10^{-2} Sv^{-1}, but does not significantly change the values of the tissue weighting factors.

(98) If the equivalent dose is fairly uniform over the whole body, it is possible to obtain the probability of fatal cancer associated with that effective dose from the nominal fatality probability coefficient. If the distribution of equivalent dose is non-uniform, this use of the nominal coefficient will be less accurate because the tissue weighting factors include allowances for non-fatal and hereditary conditions. For example, the contribution of fatalities from the equivalent dose in the lung will be underestimated by about 25%, and the contribution from the skin and thyroid will be overestimated by a factor of about 3. If the tissue equivalent doses are known, the nominal fatality probability coefficients for the individual tissues and organ can be used, but the difference between the two methods will not be significant because the individual tissue coefficients are not known with sufficient accuracy. The necessary data for both methods are provided in Table 4. As an approximation for a wide range of distributions of equivalent dose, the non-fatal somatic detriment adds about 20–30% to the fatal detriment.

4. THE CONCEPTUAL FRAMEWORK OF RADIOLOGICAL PROTECTION

Chapter 4 deals with the general policy of radiological protection. It introduces the idea of source-related and individual-related assessments. It outlines the basic system of protection for occupational, medical, and public exposures and distinguishes between a "practice", which causes exposures to radiation, and "intervention", which decreases exposures.

4.1. The Basic Framework

(99) Everyone in the world is exposed to radiation from natural and artificial sources. Any realistic system of radiological protection must therefore have a clearly defined scope if it is not to apply to the whole of mankind's activities. It also has to cover, in a consistent way, a very wide range of circumstances.

(100) The basic framework of radiological protection necessarily has to include social as well as scientific judgements, because the primary aim of radiological protection is to provide an appropriate standard of protection for man without unduly limiting the beneficial practices giving rise to radiation exposure. Furthermore, it must be presumed that even small radiation doses may produce some deleterious health effects. Since there are thresholds for deterministic effects, it is possible to avoid them by restricting the doses to individuals. On the other hand, stochastic effects cannot be completely avoided because no threshold can be invoked for them. The Commission's basic framework is intended to prevent the occurrence of deterministic effects, by keeping doses below the relevant thresholds, and to ensure that all reasonable steps are taken to reduce the induction of stochastic effects.

(101) Most decisions about human activities are based on an implicit form of balancing benefits against costs and disadvantages, leading to the conclusion that a particular course of action or practice either is, or is not, worthwhile. Less commonly, it is also recognised that the conduct of a practice should be adjusted to maximise the net benefit to the individual or to society. This is not a simple process because the objectives

of the individual and society may not coincide. In radiological protection, as in other areas, it is becoming possible to formalise and quantify procedures that help in reaching these decisions. In doing so, attention has to be paid, not only to the advantages and disadvantages for society as a whole, but also to the protection of individuals. When the benefits and detriments do not have the same distribution through the population, there is bound to be some inequity. Serious inequity can be avoided by the attention paid to the protection of individuals. It must also be recognised that many current practices give rise to doses that will be received in the future, sometimes the far future. These future doses should be taken into account in the protection of both populations and individuals, although not necessarily on the same basis as is used for current doses. Current practices may also give rise to a probability, but not a certainty, that exposures will occur. The probability of incurring the exposures is then important, in addition to the magnitude of the exposures.

(102) To clarify the way in which the Commission has developed its recommendations, it is convenient to think of the processes causing human exposures as a network of events and situations. Each part of the network starts from a source. This term is used by the Commission to indicate the source of an exposure, not necessarily a physical source of radiation. Thus the source of occupational exposures in a hospital might be the x-ray units, rather than the anodes which are the physical source of the x rays. When radioactive materials are released to the environment as waste, the installation as a whole might be regarded as the source. Radiation or radioactive material then passes through environmental pathways, which may be simple in a workplace, but very complex in the natural environment, with some pathways being common to many sources. Eventually, individuals, possibly many individuals, are exposed as a result of a single original source. Since there can be many sources, some individuals will be exposed to radiation from more than one of them. If natural sources are included, all individuals are exposed to radiation from at least a few sources.

(103) Fortunately, it is rarely necessary to treat this network as a single entity. Provided that the individual doses are well below the threshold for deterministic effects, the contribution to an individual dose from a single source has an effect that is independent of the doses from other sources. For many purposes, each source, or group of sources, can then be treated on its own. Each individual, however, is exposed as a result of several sources. It follows that assessments of the effectiveness of protection can be related to the source giving rise to the individual doses (source-related) or related to the individual dose received by a person from all the relevant sources (individual-related).

(104) Source-related assessments make it possible to judge whether a source is likely to bring benefits sufficient to outweigh any disadvantages that it may have, and whether all reasonable steps have been taken to reduce the radiation exposures that it will cause. The source-related assessment will take account of the magnitude and the probability of occurrence of individual doses attributable to that source, and of the number of individuals so exposed, but will not consider the additional contributions from other sources.

(105) It will therefore be necessary also to consider an individual-related assessment of the total doses in individuals from all the relevant sources, in order to determine whether any individual has too high a probability of stochastic effects and whether any individual dose approaches one of the thresholds for deterministic effects.

(106) Some human activities increase the overall exposure to radiation, either by

introducing whole new blocks of sources, pathways, and individuals, or by modifying the network of pathways from existing sources to man and thus increasing the exposure of individuals or the number of individuals exposed. The Commission calls these human activities "practices". Other human activities can decrease the overall exposure by influencing the existing form of the network. These activities may remove existing sources, modify pathways, or reduce the number of exposed individuals. The Commission describes all these activities as "intervention".

(107) The steps needed to restrict the exposure of individuals, either in the control of a practice or by intervention, can be taken by applying action at any point in the network linking the sources to the individuals. The action may be applied to the source, to the environment, or to the individual. Actions that can be applied at the source will be the least disruptive. They can be made as effective as is required, unless they fail as the result of an accident. They influence all the pathways and individuals associated with that source. In the extreme case, the action may be to avoid the use of the source. Where available, controls applied at the source are to be preferred. Actions applied to the environment or to individuals are more obtrusive and may have social disadvantages, not all of which are foreseeable. Their effectiveness will be limited because they apply only to some of the pathways and individuals.

(108) The Commission's system of protection is intended to be as general as possible, partly for consistency and partly to avoid changes of policy resulting from the demarcation of different situations. However, the various types of exposure and the distinction between practices and intervention give rise to different degrees of controllability and thus influence the judgements about the reasonableness of the various control procedures.

(109) The Commission uses a division into three types of exposure: occupational exposure, which is the exposure incurred at work, and principally as a result of work; medical exposure, which is principally the exposure of persons as part of their diagnosis or treatment; and public exposure, which comprises all other exposures. More detailed descriptions are given in Chapter 5.

(110) In the control of occupational exposure, it is usually possible to apply controls at all three points: at the source, by fixing its characteristics and its immediate shielding and containment; in the environment, by ventilation or additional shielding; and at the individual, by requiring working practices and the use of protective clothing and equipment. Not all these levels of control are needed all the time. In medical exposures, the controls are also applied at all three points, but mainly as part of the primary function of diagnosis or treatment, rather than as part of a separate system of protection. In public exposure, the controls should be applied at the source. Only if these cannot be made effective should controls be applied to the environment or to individuals.

(111) The appropriate control measures also depend on whether they are to be applied to a practice causing exposures or to intervention aimed at reducing exposures. In the case of a new practice, there is the option of accepting the practice, as proposed or with modifications, or of rejecting it outright. Existing practices can be reviewed in the light of new information or changed standards of protection and, at least in principle, can be withdrawn; but the sources and pathways that they involve may persist. Any further changes then require intervention. Accidents, once they have occurred, give rise to situations in which the only available action is some form of intervention. In practices and in intervention, it will often be virtually certain that exposures will occur and their magnitude will be predictable, albeit with some degree of uncertainty. Sometimes, how-

ever, there will be a potential for exposure, but no certainty that it will occur. The Commission calls such exposures "potential exposures". It is often possible to apply some degree of control to both the probability and the magnitude of potential exposures.

4.2. The System of Radiological Protection

(112) The system of radiological protection recommended by the Commission for proposed and continuing practices is based on the following general principles. Details of the system in relation to practices are given in Chapter 5. The system for intervention is discussed in the next paragraph and in Chapter 6.

(a) No practice involving exposures to radiation should be adopted unless it produces sufficient benefit to the exposed individuals or to society to offset the radiation detriment it causes. (The justification of a practice.)

(b) In relation to any particular source within a practice, the magnitude of individual doses, the number of people exposed, and the likelihood of incurring exposures where these are not certain to be received should all be kept as low as reasonably achievable, economic and social factors being taken into account. This procedure should be constrained by restrictions on the doses to individuals (dose constraints), or the risks to individuals in the case of potential exposures (risk constraints), so as to limit the inequity likely to result from the inherent economic and social judgements. (The optimisation of protection.)

(c) The exposure of individuals resulting from the combination of all the relevant practices should be subject to dose limits, or to some control of risk in the case of potential exposures. These are aimed at ensuring that no individual is exposed to radiation risks that are judged to be unacceptable from these practices in any normal circumstances. Not all sources are susceptible of control by action at the source and it is necessary to specify the sources to be included as relevant before selecting a dose limit. (Individual dose and risk limits.)

(113) The system of radiological protection recommended by the Commission for intervention is based on the following general principles.

(a) The proposed intervention should do more good than harm, i.e. the reduction in detriment resulting from the reduction in dose should be sufficient to justify the harm and the costs, including social costs, of the intervention.

(b) The form, scale, and duration of the intervention should be optimised so that the net benefit of the reduction of dose, i.e. the benefit of the reduction in radiation detriment, less the detriment associated with the intervention, should be maximised.

Dose limits do not apply in the case of intervention (see paragraph 131). Principles (a) and (b) can lead to intervention levels which give guidance to the situations in which intervention is appropriate. There will be some level of projected dose above which, because of serious deterministic effects, intervention will almost always be justified.

(114) Any system of protection should include an overall assessment of its effectiveness in practice. This should be based on the distribution of doses achieved and on an appraisal of the steps taken to limit the probability of potential exposures. It is important that the basic principles should be treated as a coherent system. No one part should be taken in isolation. In particular, mere compliance with the dose limits is not a sufficient demonstration of satisfactory performance.

4.3. Radiological Protection in Proposed and Continuing Practices

4.3.1. *The justification of a practice*

(115) Decisions concerning the adoption and continuation of any human activity involve a choice between possible options and are often carried out in two stages. The first stage is the examination of each option separately in order to identify those options which can be expected to do more good than harm. This provides a "short list" from which the preferred option can then be selected. The second stage, the final selection, will often involve the replacement of one existing practice by another. The net benefit of the change will then be the relevant feature rather than the net benefit of each option separately. The Commission recommends that, when practices involving exposure, or potential exposure, to radiation are being considered, the radiation detriment should be explicitly included in the process of choice. The detriment to be considered is not confined to that associated with the radiation—it includes other detriments and the costs of the practice. Often, the radiation detriment will be a small part of the total. The justification of a practice thus goes far beyond the scope of radiological protection. It is for these reasons that the Commission limits its use of the term justification to the first of the above stages, i.e. it requires only that the net benefit be positive. To search for the best of all the available options is usually a task beyond the responsibility of radiological protection agencies.

(116) The process of justification is required, not only when a new practice is being introduced, but also when existing practices are being reviewed in the light of new information about their efficacy or consequences. If such a review indicates that a practice could no longer be claimed to produce sufficient benefit to offset the total detriment, withdrawal of the practice should be considered. This option should be treated in the same way as the justification of a new practice, but it must be remembered that the disadvantages of withdrawing a well-established practice may be more obvious than the advantages of introducing a comparable new one and withdrawal of the practice may not result in the withdrawal of all the associated sources of exposure. Preventing the further extension of an existing practice that is no longer justified may sometimes be a reasonable compromise, but will introduce an anomaly between the past and the present and will not always be seen as logical.

4.3.2. *The optimisation of protection*

(117) Once a practice has been justified and adopted, it is necessary to consider how best to use resources in reducing the radiation risks to individuals and the population. The broad aim should be to ensure that the magnitude of the individual doses, the number of people exposed, and the likelihood of incurring exposures where these are not certain to be received, are all kept as low as reasonably achievable, economic and social factors being taken into account. Consideration has to be given to any interaction between these various quantities. If the next step of reducing the detriment can be achieved only with a deployment of resources that is seriously out of line with the consequent reduction, it is not in society's interest to take that step, provided that individuals have been adequately protected. The protection can then be said to be optimised and the exposures to be as low as reasonably achievable, economic and social factors having been taken into account. The procedure should also be applied when an existing practice is being reviewed.

(118) These considerations are complicated by the interaction between the various

factors to be included, and the methods for dealing with them are diverse. They range from simple common sense to complex techniques of cost-benefit analysis or multi-attribute analysis. In the Commission's view, all these techniques are aids to deciding when sufficient effort has been applied to the reduction of the detriment associated with a practice or with an identifiable component of a practice. Except when dealing with potential exposures, it is appropriate to use the effective dose as a surrogate for detriment to an individual, because the weighting factors used in calculating the effective dose take account of the whole detriment to the health of individuals and their descendants, not only the fatal detriment. The collective effective dose is an adequate representation of the collective detriment. For potential exposures, the situation is more complicated. (See Section 4.3.4.)

(119) The judgements involved in optimising protection are not purely quantitative—they involve preferences between detriments of different kinds and between the deployment of resources and health effects. Guidance on the necessary techniques has already been published by the Commission in *Publication 37* (1983) and *Publication 55* (1989).

(120) The process of optimising protection should be carefully structured. It is essentially source-related and should first be applied at the design stage of any project. It is here that dose reductions are most likely to be achievable in cost-effective ways. In achieving a design optimised for protection, designers should take account of, and influence, the way the plant or equipment will subsequently be used, although their information and influence on these future operational aspects may be limited. They may also wish to take account of the substantial advantages offered by engineering standardisation. At the design stage, therefore, the process of optimisation of protection will have some generic aspects. Further optimisation of protection should be carried out at the operational level. Operational optimisation is usually informal, involving common-sense changes in procedures, but is often very effective.

(121) Most of the methods used in the optimisation of protection tend to emphasise the benefits and detriments to society and the whole exposed population. The benefits and detriments are unlikely to be distributed through society in the same way. Optimisation of protection may thus introduce a substantial inequity between one individual and another. This inequity can be limited by incorporating source-related restrictions on individual dose into the process of optimisation. The Commission calls these source-related restrictions dose constraints, previously called upper bounds. They form an integral part of the optimisation of protection. For potential exposures, the corresponding concept is the risk constraint. The choice of constraints depends on the circumstances and is discussed further in Chapter 5.

4.3.3. *Individual dose limits*

(122) If the procedures of justification of practices and of optimisation of protection have been conducted effectively, there will be few cases where limits on individual dose will have to be applied. However, such limits provide a clearly defined boundary for these more subjective procedures and prevent excessive individual detriment, which might result from a combination of practices. The Commission's dose limits should be applied only in the control of practices.

(123) It is the Commission's intention to choose the values of dose limits so that any continued exposure just above the dose limits would result in additional risks from the defined practices that could reasonably be described as "unacceptable" in normal circumstances. Thus the definition and choice of dose limits involve social judgements.

These judgements are difficult, partly because the dose limit has to be set at a defined value and there is no discontinuity in the scale of acceptability. For agents like ionising radiation, for which no threshold can be assumed in the dose–response relationship for some of the consequences of exposure, this difficulty is inescapable and the choice of limits cannot be based on health considerations alone.

(124) In practice, several misconceptions have arisen about the definition and function of dose limits. In the first place, the dose limit is widely, but erroneously, regarded as a line of demarcation between "safe" and "dangerous". Secondly, it is also widely, and also erroneously, seen as the most simple and effective way of keeping exposures low and forcing improvements. Thirdly, it is commonly seen as the sole measure of the stringency of a system of protection. These misconceptions are, to some extent, strengthened by the incorporation of dose limits into regulatory instruments. Causing a dose limit to be exceeded then becomes an infraction of the rules and sometimes a statutory offence. Against this background, it is not surprising that managements, regulatory agencies, and governments all improperly set out to apply dose limits whenever possible, even when the sources are partly, or even totally, beyond their control, and when the optimisation of protection is the more appropriate course of action.

(125) It has also become apparent that dose limits are commonly used in two very different ways. In one application, mainly related to occupational exposure, the dose limit is regarded as a limiting restriction on the design and operation of an installation. In the other way, the dose limit is used in its original function of applying controls on each individual's accumulation of dose. It will never be appropriate to apply dose limits to all types of exposure in all circumstances. In circumstances for which they were not intended, e.g. in emergencies or during special operations of considerable importance, they can often be replaced by specially developed prescriptive limits or by specified levels of dose that call for the initiation of a defined course of action. Such levels, often called action or investigation levels or, in more general cases, reference levels, provide a useful way of structuring the procedures of radiological protection.

(126) For the above reasons the Commission has had to develop a more complex approach to dose limits. The specification of dose limits and the choice of values are discussed in Chapter 5.

4.3.4. *Potential exposures*

(127) Not all exposures occur as forecast. There may be accidental departures from the planned operating procedures, or equipment may fail. Environmental changes may occur after the disposal of radioactive waste, or there may be changes in the way in which the environment is used. Such events can be foreseen and their probability of occurrence estimated, but they cannot be predicted in detail. The concept of both individual and collective detriment resulting from an exposure then has to be extended to allow for the fact that the exposure may not occur.

(128) Potential exposures need to be considered as part of the assessment of practices, but they may also lead to calls for intervention. Their implications should therefore be considered in both contexts. If the probability of occurrence of the event causing the potential exposures is fairly high, so that several such events might be expected within a year, it should be assumed that the doses resulting from the event will certainly occur.

(129) Dose limits do not apply directly to potential exposures. Ideally, they should be supplemented by risk limits, which take account of both the probability of incurring a dose and the detriment associated with that dose if it were to be received. However, risk

limits differ from dose limits in that the probability of occurrence and the magnitude of the potential exposure cannot be determined—they can only be inferred from an assessment of future scenarios. Furthermore, a potential exposure may become a real exposure and may then call for intervention. The problems are discussed further in Section 5.6.

4.4. Radiological Protection by Intervention

(130) In some situations, the sources, the pathways, and the exposed individuals are already in place when the decisions about control measures are being considered. Sometimes, the new control procedures can be achieved as part of a review of the original practice, but, more commonly, they will constitute intervention. An important group of such situations is that involving exposure to natural sources of radiation. Accidents and emergencies will have been considered as sources of potential exposure when dealing with practices, but if they occur, they may call for intervention. All these cases are dealt with in Chapter 6.

(131) In most situations, intervention cannot be applied at the source and has to be applied in the environment and to individuals' freedom of action. The countermeasures forming a programme of intervention, which always have some disadvantages, should be justified in the sense that they should do more good than harm. Their form, scale and duration should then be optimised so as to maximise the net benefit. The dose limits recommended by the Commission are intended for use in the control of practices. The use of these dose limits, or of any other pre-determined dose limits, as the basis for deciding on intervention might involve measures that would be out of all proportion to the benefit obtained and would then conflict with the principle of justification. The Commission therefore recommends against the application of dose limits for deciding on the need for, or scope of, intervention. Nevertheless, at some level of dose, approaching that which would cause serious deterministic effects, some kind of intervention will become almost mandatory.

4.5. The Assessment of the Effectiveness of a System of Protection

(132) When establishing that a system of protection is satisfactory, it is necessary to assess the overall effectiveness of the system. It is not appropriate merely to examine its component parts separately. When dealing with proposed or continuing practices, the expected or observed distributions of individual doses and the collective effective dose from defined operations should be considered. Comparisons between comparable operations and trends with time will often indicate the possibility of improvements. The assessment is more difficult for potential exposures because it is necessary to depend on an examination of the procedures for estimating the probability of the exposures. The probabilities cannot be directly determined. For intervention, including that resulting from accidents, the assessment should concentrate on the effectiveness of the forward planning and, retrospectively, on the effectiveness of the action taken in particular cases.

5. THE SYSTEM OF PROTECTION FOR PROPOSED AND CONTINUING PRACTICES

Chapter 5 indicates how the Commission develops the concepts described in Chapter 4 in the contexts of Occupational Exposure (the exposure of people at work), Medical Exposure (the exposure of people as part of their medical diagnosis or treatment), and

Public Exposure (all other exposures to radiation). It relates to practices, which cause exposure to radiation, and excludes intervention. It sets out the main structure of the recommended control procedures and, where relevant, defines the scope and recommended values of dose limits.

(133) The basic policies underlying the system of protection recommended by the Commission and described in Chapter 4 are developed in this chapter for application to practices. The chapter is subdivided to take account of the several types of exposure identified in Chapter 4, namely Occupational Exposure, Medical Exposure, and Public Exposure. There are many circumstances in which these types of exposure are best treated and discussed separately, as in this Chapter. Nevertheless, this separation is not always appropriate. For example, all types of exposure resulting from a practice have to be considered together in the justification of that practice. The justification of a practice has therefore been discussed fully in Chapter 4. However, some additional aspects of justification relating to medical practices are dealt with in Section 5.4.1. There are also situations in which decisions about public exposure interact with occupational exposures. These interactive situations are discussed in Section 5.7. The practical arrangements suggested for implementing the system of protection are discussed in Chapter 7.

5.1. Types of Exposure

5.1.1. *Occupational exposure*

(134) The Commission has noted the conventional definition of occupational exposure to any hazardous agent as including all exposures incurred at work, regardless of their source. However, because of the ubiquity of radiation, the direct application of this definition to radiation would mean that all workers should be subject to a regime of radiological protection. The Commission therefore limits its use of the phrase "occupational exposure (to radiation)" to exposures incurred at work as the result of situations that can reasonably be regarded as being the responsibility of the operating management.

(135) Of the components of exposure to natural sources, those due to potassium-40 in the body, cosmic rays at ground level, and radionuclides in the earth's crust are all outside any reasonable scope of control. Only radon in workplaces and work with materials containing natural radionuclides can reasonably be regarded as the responsibility of the operating management. Furthermore, there is some exposure to radon in all workplaces, and it is important not to require the use of a formal system of separate decisions to exempt each individual workplace where controls are not needed. They should be excluded from the control of occupational exposure by some general system. Considerable knowledge and judgement is needed to define such a system. The Commission recommends that exposure to radon and the handling of materials containing traces of natural radionuclides should be regarded as excluded from occupational exposure and treated separately, unless the relevant regulatory agency has ruled otherwise, either in a defined geographical area or for defined practices.

(136) To provide some practical guidance, the Commission recommends that there should be a requirement to include exposures to natural sources as part of occupational exposure only in the following cases:

(a) Operations in workplaces where the regulatory agency has declared that radon needs attention and has identified the relevant workplaces.

   (b) Operations with and storage of materials not usually regarded as radioactive, but which contain significant traces of natural radionuclides and which have been identified by the regulatory agency.

   (c) Operation of jet aircraft.

   (d) Space flight.

The definition of quantified specifications for cases (a) and (b) will depend on the local circumstances; but, as a very general guide, operations in spas, in most uranium mines, including open-cast mines, in many other underground mines and caves, and in some other underground workplaces are likely to constitute examples of case (a). Case (c) will relate principally to the aircraft crew, but attention should also be paid to groups such as couriers who fly more often than other passengers. Case (d) relates to very few individuals and will not be discussed further here.

   (137) It is also necessary to consider how exposures to natural sources should be dealt with in workplaces where there is already a need for controls on the exposures directly associated with the work. It will be sufficient to take account of the exposures to natural sources if, and only if, they would be controlled in their own right as indicated in the previous paragraph. Elsewhere, they need not be included in radiation monitoring results, or in statistical reports of occupational exposures.

   (138) Any exposure at work (excluding any medical exposure at work) as a result of artificial sources in, or associated with, the workplace should be included in occupational exposure, unless the sources have formally been excluded from regulatory control or exempted from the relevant aspects of regulatory control by the regulatory agency. Guidance on exclusion and exemption is given in Section 7.8.

5.1.2. *Medical exposure*

   (139) Medical exposure is confined to exposures incurred by individuals as part of their own medical diagnosis or treatment and to exposures (other than occupational) incurred knowingly and willingly by individuals helping in the support and comfort of patients undergoing diagnosis or treatment. Exposure of an individual to other sources, such as stray radiation from the diagnosis or treatment of other persons, is not included in medical exposure. Nor is any occupational exposure of staff. Exposures incurred by volunteers as part of a programme of biomedical research are also dealt with in this document on the same basis as medical exposure.

5.1.3. *Public exposure*

   (140) Public exposure encompasses all exposures other than occupational and medical exposures. The component of public exposure due to natural sources is by far the largest, but this provides no justification for reducing the attention paid to smaller, but more readily controlled, exposures to artificial sources.

5.2. The Application of the System of Protection

   (141) The system of radiological protection described in Chapter 4 can usually be applied in much the same way in all types of exposure. Where there are significant differences, these are discussed in the following Sections. To some extent, different methods of application are needed for potential exposures, which are discussed separately in Section 5.6. Intervention is discussed in Chapter 6.

(142) It is necessary to consider the implications for radiological protection of different coefficients linking effective dose and detriment for different ages and sexes. These differences result from the effect of competing causes of death and the different intrinsic sensitivity of some tissues, notably the breast. However, as indicated in Section 3.5, reflecting these differences would have only a small effect on the definition of effective dose and on the nominal probability coefficient. In addition, many of the most effective methods of controlling exposures are applied without reference to the age and sex of those exposed, so it is desirable to set limits and to optimise protection in ways that are independent of both age and sex.

(143) The dose limits recommended in the following sections apply only to the sum of dose contribution from a relevant set of exposures and not to those from all sources of radiation. Because the identification of the relevant dose contributions cannot easily be generalised, the details are given in the following sections. However, in all cases the limits apply to the sum of all relevant doses from external exposure in the specified periods and the committed doses from intakes during the same periods.

5.3. The System of Protection in Occupational Exposure

5.3.1. *The optimisation of protection in occupational exposure*

(144) An important feature of optimisation is the choice of dose constraints, the source-related values of individual dose used to limit the range of options considered in the procedure of optimisation. For many types of occupation, it is possible to reach conclusions about the level of individual doses likely to be incurred in well-managed operations. This information can then be used to establish a dose constraint for that type of occupation. In the Commission's view, the class of occupation should be specified in fairly broad terms, such as work in x-ray diagnostic departments, the routine operation of nuclear power plants, or the inspection and maintenance of nuclear power plants. Limits prescribed by regulatory agencies and restrictions applied by managements to specific operations as part of the day-to-day control of exposures are not constraints in the sense used here. In general, these limits and restrictions should be established on the basis of the results of optimisation. More information is given in Section 7.3.1.

(145) It will usually be appropriate for dose constraints to be fixed at the national or local level. When using a dose constraint, a designer should specify the sources to which it is linked so as to avoid confusion with other sources to which the workforce might be concurrently exposed.

(146) The optimisation of protection should, in principle, take account of both actual and potential exposures. However, the techniques for potential exposures are less well developed and the decisions about potential exposures often have no implications for actual exposures. They can then be dealt with separately. (See Section 5.6.)

5.3.2. *Dose limits in occupational exposure*

(147) Dose limits are needed as part of the control of occupational exposure both to impose a limit on the choice of dose constraints (to cover the occasional case where the same individual is employed on several tasks each with its own constraint) and to provide a protection against errors of judgement in the application of optimisation. In practice, occupational dose limits are applied to all occupational exposure as defined in Section 5.1.1, including that resulting from minor mishaps and misjudgements in operations and

from maintenance and decommissioning in circumstances not necessarily envisaged by the designers. This is an extension of the Commission's previous concept of dose limits and represents a significant increase in the stringency of the Commission's recommendations, regardless of any change in the magnitude of the limits.

(148) The basis of choosing a limit on the risks to which an individual may be subjected has always been difficult to specify. In its 1977 recommendations for dose limits applied to occupational exposure, the Commission attempted to use a comparison with the rates of accidental death in industries not associated with radiation. These comparisons are not altogether satisfactory for a number of reasons. For example, standards of industrial safety are neither constant nor uniform world-wide; the mortality data relate to averages over whole industries, whereas dose limits apply to individuals; the quantitative comparisons were limited to mortality data although the inclusion of non-fatal conditions on both sides of the comparison would have led to less restrictive dose limits; and, finally, there are few grounds for believing that society expects the same standard of safety across a wide range of industries.

(149) The Commission has now adopted a more comprehensive approach. The aim is to establish, for a defined set of practices, a level of dose above which the consequences for the individual would be widely regarded as unacceptable. For this purpose, the limiting dose can be expressed as a lifetime dose received uniformly over the working life, or as an annual dose received every year of work, without prejudice to the way in which the dose limit is finally specified. In the past, the Commission has used the attributable probability of either death or severe hereditary conditions as the basis for judging the consequences of an exposure. This quantity is still a major factor, but is no longer regarded by the Commission as sufficient to describe the detriment. Other factors have been considered in the definition of detriment (see Section 3.3). They include the length of life lost due to an attributable death and the incidence of non-fatal conditions.

(150) In principle, a single index representing the detriment, as now defined, could be used to quantify the consequences of an exposure, but it is extremely difficult to judge the implications of a stated detriment expressed as a single aggregated index, and thus to judge its tolerability. The Commission has found it useful to use three words to indicate the degree of tolerability of an exposure (or risk). They are necessarily subjective in character and must be interpreted in relation to the type and source of the exposure under consideration. The first word is "unacceptable", which is used to indicate that the exposure would, in the Commission's view, not be acceptable on any reasonable basis in the normal operation of any practice of which the use was a matter of choice. Such exposures might have to be accepted in abnormal situations, such as those during accidents. Exposures that are not unacceptable are then subdivided into those that are "tolerable", meaning that they are not welcome but can reasonably be tolerated, and "acceptable", meaning that they can be accepted without further improvement i.e. when the protection has been optimised. In this framework, a dose limit represents a selected boundary in the region between "unacceptable" and "tolerable" for the situation to which the dose limit is to apply, i.e. for the control of practices. Levels of exposure that are regarded as unacceptable in this context may still be tolerable in other contexts; if, for example, they can be reduced only by abandoning a desirable practice e.g., space missions.

(151) In order to provide a quantitative basis for the choice of a dose limit, the Commission has taken account of a range of quantifiable factors in its approach to detriment. For none of them is it possible to establish a categorical criterion against

which to define unacceptable and tolerable, but, taken together, they provide a basis for judgement. Data on the factors considered are given in Annexes B and C.

(152) The Commission has considered these quantifiable factors by selecting several possible values of dose that might be adopted as a dose limit. These test values have been expressed as annual doses received each year over a working lifetime of 47 years. The total dose accumulated has also been considered. The relationship between annual and accumulated dose is valid for external sources of exposure and for short-lived internal sources. If the radionuclides in the body are long-lived and have long biological retention times, the dose is spread out in time and may not all be delivered during the lifetime of the individual. The following assessment then somewhat overestimates the consequences of internal exposures expressed in terms of the 50-year committed equivalent dose.

(153) The consequences of the continued uniform exposure to each of the test values in turn are evaluated. A view is then reached as to which value gives rise to a combination of consequences that is judged to be just short of unacceptable, i.e. just tolerable. This value is then selected as the dose limit. This approach is inevitably subjective, but it makes it possible to consider a wide range of inter-related factors, more properly called attributes. The attributes associated with mortality are as follows:

The lifetime attributable probability of death.

The time lost if the attributable death occurs.

The reduction of life expectancy (a combination of the first two attributes).

The annual distribution of the attributable probability of death.

The increase in the age specific mortality rate, i.e. in the probability of dying in a year at any age, conditional on reaching that age.

(154) These attributes relate to mortality. The Commission has decided to allow for morbidity due to non-fatal cancer and hereditary disorders by using the number of non-fatal conditions weighted for severity as discussed in Section 3.5, and for the period of life lost or impaired. For non-fatal cancers, this weighted number amounts to about 20% of the detriment due to fatalities. The weighted figure for hereditary conditions is very uncertain, but is estimated at about 20% of the number of fatalities for workers (about 27% for the whole population). These contributions are included separately in the following comparisons. They are also summed to give an indication of the aggregated detriment.

(155) The test values of annual effective dose selected for review as a possible basis for the dose limit are 10 mSv, 20 mSv, 30 mSv, and 50 mSv, corresponding approximately to lifetime doses of 0.5 Sv, 1.0 Sv, 1.4 Sv, and 2.4 Sv, given that the annual doses are received every working year. It is implicit in this approach that it is not appropriate to make a decision on the basis of a single attribute. Combinations of attributes should be considered and a judgement should be made on the basis of the whole structure. Annex C provides the necessary age specific calculations. The results are adequately representative of the wider range of populations mentioned in Annex B. The attributes for the test values of annual effective dose are shown in Table 5.

(156) The first combination reviewed is that of the probability of an attributable fatal cancer and the average period of life lost if the attributable fatality occurs. For an annual dose, received every working year, this combination can be expressed as a lifetime probability of losing, on average, a stated period of time. This period is almost independent of the annual dose, since, at low doses, it depends only on the time of the

Table 5. Attributes of detriment due to exposure of the working population[1]

	10	20	30	50	50 (1977 data)
Annual effective dose (mSv)	10	20	30	50	50 (1977 data)
Approximate lifetime dose (Sv)	0.5	1.0	1.4	2.4	2.4
Probability of attributable death (%)	1.8	3.6	5.3	8.6	2.9
Weighted contribution from non-fatal cancer (%)[2]	0.4	0.7	1.1	1.7	—
Weighted contribution from hereditary effects (%)[2]	0.4	0.7	1.1	1.7	1.2
Aggregated detriment (%)[3]	2.5	5	7.5	12	
Time lost due to an attributable death given that it occurs (y)	13	13	13	13	10–15
Mean loss of life expectancy at age 18 years (y)	0.2	0.5	0.7	1.1	0.3–0.5

[1] The values are all derived from Annex C (see paragraph 155); in Annex B, which deals with a wider range of populations, a somewhat higher estimate is given for the time lost due to an attributable death.
[2] Weighted for severity and loss of lifetime.
[3] The sum of the probability of attributable fatal cancer or equivalent detriment (rounded).

attributable death, not on its probability. For the combination of an additive risk projection model for leukaemia and a multiplicative model for other cancers, the loss is slightly less than 13 years. For the additive model, the loss is slightly less than 20 years. Another attribute, itself an aggregation of these data, is the mean loss of life expectancy at age 18 years as a result of subsequent occupational exposure.

(157) In Table 5, results derived from the data available in 1977 for an annual dose of 50 mSv over 40 years are included for comparison. It should be recognised that these numbers were not used as the basis for selection of the dose limit at that time. As indicated in paragraph 148 the selection of the 1977 limit was made on an entirely different basis (comparing the average fatal cancer risk in radiation work with the fatality risk in "safe" non-radiation occupations and assuming a ratio of 10:1 between the maximum and the average risk). Since the Commission no longer considers that method satisfactory, the 1977 results in the table give little guidance for the present choice of dose limit and have not been used for that purpose.

(158) The way in which the annual probability of attributable death varies with time is also of interest and is shown in Figure 2. The combined effect of latency and the extended period of exposure is to produce a distribution sharply peaked in time at older ages for both the additive risk projection model and the multiplicative risk projection model. The curves are for women, but those for men are very similar. The age of maximum (unconditional) annual probability of attributable death following the exposure of a population of equal numbers of men and women over a whole working lifetime occurs at 68 years for the additive model and 78 years for the multiplicative model. This age is almost independent of the annual dose. The term "unconditional" is used to indicate that the probability is not conditional on reaching the age for which the probability is quoted. The conditional probability continues to rise indefinitely.

(159) The changes in the age-specific mortality rate (roughly the probability of dying within a year conditional on reaching the beginning of that year) are best shown graphically. The data are presented in Annex C (Figure C-9). Even for a continued annual dose of 50 mSv, the changes in mortality rate are small compared with the differences in mortality rate between men and women.

(160) Before any attempt is made to choose a dose limit from this quantitative material, it is necessary to remember that the Commission's aim at this stage is to reach a judgement about a level of dose that would reasonably be regarded as being only just short of unacceptable in the control of practices. The levels of dose actually achieved are

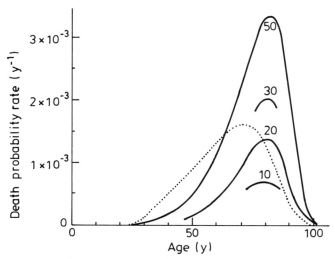

Fig. 2. The unconditional death probability rate (the attributable death age probability density normalised for lifetime risk) for exposure from age 18 to age 65 y. The curves are for females and for present risk estimates.
····· Additive risk projection model (50 mSv y^{-1})
———— Multiplicative risk projection model (showing various annual doses in mSv)

not relevant for the purpose of this assessment. The data are expressed in terms of an annual dose over a full working lifetime of 47 years. The form in which the dose limits are best expressed for practical application is discussed later in this section.

(161) The first conclusion drawn by the Commission is that there is no need to extend the range of test doses to be considered in the choice of a dose limit for occupational exposure. The second is that the results indicate that a regular annual dose of 50 mSv, corresponding to a lifetime effective dose of 2.4 Sv, is probably too high, and would be regarded by many as being clearly so. In particular, the reduction of life expectancy at this level (1.1 years) and the fact that there would be a probability exceeding 8% that the radiation hazards in a worker's occupation would be the cause of his death, albeit at a late age, would be widely seen as excessive for a group of occupations many of which are of recent origin and should therefore be setting an example.

(162) On the basis of the data presented above, the Commission has reached the judgement that its dose limit should be set in such a way and at such a level that the total effective dose received in a full working life would be prevented from exceeding about 1 Sv received moderately uniformly year by year and that the application of its system of radiological protection should be such that this figure would only rarely be approached. The final choice of limits and the way in which they should be expressed are influenced by the way in which the limits will be applied in practice. The need to ensure that the limits provide protection against deterministic effects also has to be taken into account.

(163) At the levels of dose incurred in normal situations, excluding doses to the patient in radiotherapy, the control of stochastic effects could be based on the dose accumulated over periods of many years. However, such long control periods can be misused by allowing a rapid accumulation of doses and intakes near the start of a control period in the expectation, not always realised, of smaller doses later in the period. Flexibility of this kind also weakens the emphasis on achieving the control of exposures by design, transferring the emphasis to operational controls.

(164) In recent years, the Commission has recommended a rigid control period of one year: i.e., it has recommended that the effective dose from sources of radiation external to the body and committed by intakes of radioactive substances into the body should be controlled over each year, with no credit taken for any earlier years of low effective dose or intake. This system is very inflexible, and alternatives have been considered.

(165) It has sometimes been suggested that the dose limits for occupational exposure might include a limit on the lifetime effective dose. The Commission sees difficulties in the practical application of lifetime limits. One of these relates to the interpretation of the limit for a worker who is employed in work involving significant occupational exposure for only part of his working life. Decisions have also to be taken about the long-term future employment of workers who exceed the lifetime limit. Short-term limits would also be needed because the Commission's risk estimates are derived for doses distributed fairly uniformly over the occupational age range. Because of these difficulties and the points made in paragraph 163, the Commission does not recommend the use of lifetime limits.

(166) It has also been suggested that flexibility might be provided by setting the limit in the form of the total dose accumulated over a period of a few years, while retaining an annual limit higher than the annual average over the longer period. This would pose some practical problems of the same type as those arising from a lifetime limit, but they would be much less severe. The Commission believes that a period of five years would adequately limit the severity of these difficulties, and would also provide sufficient flexibility. For workers on short-term contracts, the regulatory agency might consider an averaging period not exceeding the period of the contract of employment. The Commission recommends a limit on effective dose of 20 mSv per year, averaged over 5 years (100 mSv in 5 years), with the further provision that the effective dose should not exceed 50 mSv in any single year. The 5-year period would have to be defined by the regulatory agency, e.g. as discrete 5-year calendar periods. The Commission would not expect the period to be introduced and then applied retrospectively. It is implicit in these recommended dose limits that the dose constraint for optimisation should not exceed 20 mSv in a year.

(167) However the control period is defined, the Commission recommends that, following a control period in which the exposure of the individual has exceeded a dose limit, there need be no special restriction applied to the exposure of an individual. Such events should call for a thorough examination, usually by the regulatory agency, of the design and operational aspects of protection in the installation concerned, rather than for restrictions or penalties applied to the exposed individual. If the dose is unknown, or is thought to be high, referral to a physician should be considered.

(168) The recommended limits should apply to all forms of occupational exposure as defined in Section 5.1.1, unless special provisions have been made by the regulatory agency. Because of the difficulties of responding rapidly to an increase in stringency in operations on plant and equipment already in existence, the Commission recognises that regulatory agencies may wish to make temporary use of higher dose limits. Such arrangements should be regarded as transient.

(169) The dose limit forms only a part of the system of protection aimed at achieving levels of dose that are as low as reasonably achievable, economic and social factors being taken into account. It is not to be seen as a target. It represents, in the Commission's view, the point at which regular, extended, deliberate, occupational exposure can reasonably be regarded as only just tolerable.

(170) The Commission's multi-attribute approach to the selection of dose limits

necessarily includes social judgements applied to the many attributes of risk. These judgements would not necessarily be the same in all contexts and, in particular, might be different in different societies. It is for this reason that the Commission intends its guidance to be sufficiently flexible to allow for national or regional variations. In the Commission's view, however, any such variations in the protection of the most highly exposed individuals are best introduced by the use of source-related dose constraints selected by the regulatory agencies and applied in the process of the optimisation of protection rather than by the use of different dose limits.

(171) The restrictions on effective dose, even assuming that the values are at the limit for long periods, are sufficient to ensure the avoidance of deterministic effects in almost all body tissues and organs. However, there are two tissues which will not necessarily be adequately protected by a limit on effective dose, mainly in the case of external exposure. These are the lens of the eye, which makes no contribution to the effective dose, and the skin, which may well be subject to localised exposures. Separate dose limits are needed for these tissues. Internal exposures are dealt with in paragraphs 174 and 175 below.

(172) The previously recommended annual dose limit for the lens of the eye was 150 mSv. The estimated threshold of annual equivalent dose for visual impairment (cataract) was given in *Publication 41* (1984) as ">0.15 Sv" and is confirmed in Annex B. The Commission continues to recommend an annual equivalent-dose limit for the lens of the eye of 150 mSv. For external exposure to penetrating radiation over any substantial part of the whole body, the effective-dose limit will be more restrictive.

(173) For the skin, the situation is more complicated. For stochastic effects, the equivalent dose can be averaged over the whole area of the skin. The stochastic effects are expected to arise in the basal layer at a nominal depth of 7 mg cm^{-2} (range 2–10 mg cm^{-2}). Some deterministic effects also arise at the same depth, others arise in the deeper layers of the dermis (30–50 mg cm^{-2}). The limitation on the effective dose provides sufficient protection for the skin against stochastic effects. An additional limit is needed for localised exposures in order to prevent deterministic effects. The recommended annual limit is 500 mSv averaged over any 1 cm^2, regardless of the area exposed. The nominal depth is 7 mg cm^{-2}. In practice, monitoring is carried out at representative locations for external exposure and over larger areas for contamination. The guidance given in *Publication 35* (1982) on averaging areas is still valid. This limit, applied to the skin of the face, will also provide protection for the lens of the eye against localised exposures to radiation of low penetrating power such as beta particles. The same limit can be applied to all the tissues in the hands and feet.

(174) For internal exposure, annual limits on intake (ALIs) are provided by the Commission as *Publication 61* (1991) and will be based on a committed effective dose of 20 mSv. As indicated in Annex B (paragraph B52) this approach will take adequate account of any non-uniform distributions of dose within organs such as those due to hot particles. The estimated intakes may be averaged over a period of 5 years to provide some flexibility. Revised occupational limits for radon are now under review. Meanwhile the existing recommendations (*Publication 47* (1986)) remain valid.

(175) The restriction of intakes (averaged over 5 years) to the annual limit on intake will, in practice, ensure that the lifetime equivalent dose (not committed equivalent dose) in any single organ will not be such as to result in deterministic effects.

5.3.3. *The occupational exposure of women*

(176) The basis for the control of the occupational exposure of women who are not

pregnant is the same as that for men. However, if a woman is, or may be, pregnant, additional controls have to be considered to protect the unborn child. Several factors complicate this matter. The conceptus is at times more prone than the post-natal individual to deterministic injuries caused by radiation and may be more sensitive to the induction of later malignancies. It now seems clear that deterministic effects in the live-born child, including significant mental retardation, will not occur if the exposure of the mother does not exceed the dose limits now recommended for occupational exposure, regardless of the distribution of the exposures in time. Accidental higher exposures of the mother may be more damaging to the conceptus than to the mother.

(177) It is the Commission's policy that the methods of protection at work for women who may be pregnant should provide a standard of protection for any conceptus broadly comparable with that provided for members of the general public. The Commission considers that its policy will be adequately applied if the mother is exposed, prior to a declaration of pregnancy, under the system of protection recommended by the Commission, including the recommended dose limits for occupational exposure. On this basis the Commission recommends no special occupational dose limit for women in general.

(178) Once pregnancy has been declared, the conceptus should be protected by applying a supplementary equivalent-dose limit to the surface of the woman's abdomen (lower trunk) of 2 mSv for the remainder of the pregnancy and by limiting intakes of radionuclides to about 1/20 of the ALI. The Commission wishes to emphasise that the use of its system of protection, particularly the use of source-related dose constraints, will usually provide an adequate guarantee of compliance with this limit without the need for specific restrictions on the employment of pregnant women. The principal criterion will then be that the employment should be of a type that does not carry a significant probability of high accidental doses and intakes. Identification of such situations should be determined by regulatory agencies.

5.4. The System of Protection in Medical Exposure

5.4.1. *The justification of a practice in medical exposure*

(179) The justification of a practice leading to medical exposures should be dealt with in the same way as the justification of any other practice. Most of the benefits and detriment accrue to the individuals undergoing diagnosis or treatment, but account should be taken of all the resulting exposures, including the occupational and public exposures, and of any potential exposures. In the first instance, the practice should be defined in broad terms. However, each procedure, either diagnostic or therapeutic, is subject to a separate decision, so that there is an opportunity to apply a further, case-by-case, justification for each procedure. This will not be necessary for simple diagnostic procedures based on common indications, but may be important for complex investigations and for therapy. Guidance is given in *Publications 34* (1982), *44* (1985), and *52* (1987).

5.4.2. *The optimisation of protection in medical exposure*

(180) Because most procedures causing medical exposures are clearly justified and because the procedures are usually for the direct benefit of the exposed individual, less attention has been given to the optimisation of protection in medical exposure than in most other applications of radiation sources. As a result, there is considerable scope for

dose reductions in diagnostic radiology. Simple, low cost, measures are available for reducing doses without loss of diagnostic information, but the extent to which these measures are used varies widely. Doses from similar investigations cover ranges of as much as two orders of magnitude. Consideration should be given to the use of dose constraints, or investigation levels, selected by the appropriate professional or regulatory agency, for application in some common diagnostic procedures. They should be applied with flexibility to allow higher doses where indicated by sound clinical judgement.

(181) Constraints should also be considered in the optimisation of protection when the procedures are not intended to be of direct value to the exposed individual, as in scientific and clinical studies involving the exposure of volunteers.

5.4.3. *Dose limits in medical exposure*

(182) Medical exposures are usually intended to provide a direct benefit to the exposed individual. If the practice is justified and the protection optimised, the dose in the patient will be as low as is compatible with the medical purposes. Any further application of limits might be to the patient's detriment. The Commission therefore recommends that dose limits should not be applied to medical exposures. The question of dose constraints is discussed in Section 5.4.2.

(183) For reasons similar to those given in the previous paragraph, it is not appropriate to include the doses incurred by patients in the course of diagnostic examinations or therapy when considering compliance with dose limits applied to occupational or public exposures. Furthermore, each increment of dose resulting from occupational or public exposure results in an increment of detriment that is, to a large extent, unaffected by the medical doses.

5.4.4. *Medical exposure of pregnant women*

(184) As discussed in Section 3.4.4, exposure of the embryo in the first three weeks following conception is not likely to result in deterministic or stochastic effects in the liveborn child. A pregnant patient is likely to know, or at least suspect, that she is pregnant after one missed menstruation, so the necessary information on possible pregnancy can, and should, be obtained from the patient herself. If the most recent expected menstruation has been missed, and there is no other relevant information, the woman should be assumed to be pregnant. Diagnostic and therapeutic procedures causing exposures of the abdomen of women likely to be pregnant should be avoided unless there are strong clinical indications.

5.5. The System of Protection in Public Exposure

(185) The control of public exposure in all normal situations is exercised by the application of controls at the source and the controls applied in one year may lead to continuing exposures or intakes in succeeding years, for example when long lived radionuclides are to be released to the natural environment. As an alternative to the use of long-term equilibrium environmental models linking regular releases to the eventual level of individual and collective doses, the concept of dose commitment is useful. Future individual doses, more strictly the doses to typical members of a critical group, can be limited by the use of the dose commitment. If a limit is set to the effective dose commitment to a critical group from each year of practice that continues at a constant annual level, the average annual individual effective dose will never exceed that limit. If a

truncation time is used in defining the commitment, the guarantee will hold only up to the time of truncation. The collective effective dose per unit of practice can be used in the justification of a practice and in the optimisation of protection. It should be noted that part of the collective dose may be received in the distant future. If that fact is considered to be of significance in judging the importance of the detriment, the full collective dose commitment should be replaced by the collective effective dose delivered in defined periods of time.

5.5.1. *The optimisation of protection in public exposure*

(186) In practice, almost all public exposure is controlled by the procedures of constrained optimisation and the use of prescriptive limits. It is often convenient to class together individuals who form a homogeneous group with respect to their exposures to a single source. When such a group is typical of those most highly exposed by that source, it is known as a critical group. The dose constraint should be applied to the mean dose in the critical group from the source for which the protection is being optimised. Occasionally, the same group will also be critical for other sources, or, if the critical groups are different, each group may incur some dose from the sources for which it is not critical. If the exposures in any critical group are likely to approach the dose limit for public exposure (see Section 5.5.2), the constraints applied to each source must be selected to allow for any significant contribution from other sources to the exposure of the critical group.

(187) The main aim of constrained optimisation in public exposure should be to develop practical restrictions on the sources of exposure, e.g. in the form of restrictions on the release of radioactive waste to the environment.

5.5.2. *Dose limits in public exposure*

(188) With the widespread use of source-related dose constraints and practical restrictions on the sources of public exposure, generally applicable dose limits are rarely limiting in practice. However, because the constraints are source related they might, at least in principle, fail to take adequate account of the exposures from other sources. Although the Commission does not believe that this occurs to a significant extent, it continues to recommend dose limits for public exposure, if only to provide a limit on the choice of constraints.

(189) The Commission defines the scope of its dose limits for public exposure by confining it to the doses incurred as the result of practices. Doses incurred in situations where the only available protective action takes the form of intervention are excluded from the scope of the dose limits. Separate attention has to be paid to potential exposures. (See Section 5.6.) The intended emission of radionuclides from installations, including the emission of naturally occurring radionuclides from installations such as mines and waste disposal sites, should be treated as practices. The resulting doses should be subject to the dose limits. Radon in dwellings and in the open air and radioactive materials, natural or artificial, already in the environment, are examples of situations that can be influenced only by intervention. Doses from these sources are therefore outside the scope of the dose limits for public exposure. Other exposures to natural sources are also outside this scope. Radon in both existing and new dwellings is dealt with in Section 6.2.1. The conduct of intervention involves occupational exposure and should be treated accordingly.

(190) At least two approaches are possible in choosing a dose limit for public

exposure. The first is the same as that used for choosing occupational limits. Assessing the consequences is no more difficult than in the occupational case, but judging the point at which these consequences can reasonably be described as unacceptable is much more difficult. The second approach is to base the judgement on the variations in the existing level of dose from natural sources. This natural background may not be harmless, but it makes only a small contribution to the health detriment which society experiences. It may not be welcome, but the variations from place to place (excluding the large variations in the dose from radon in dwellings) can hardly be called unacceptable.

(191) The consequences of continued additional exposure giving annual effective doses in the range from 1 mSv to 5 mSv are presented in Annex C. They provide no easy basis for a judgement, but do suggest a value of the annual dose limit not much above 1 mSv. On the other hand, the data in Figure C-6 of Annex C show that, even at a continued exposure of 5 mSv y^{-1}, the change in the age specific mortality rate is very small. Excluding the very variable exposures to radon, the annual effective dose from natural sources is about 1 mSv, with values at high altitudes above sea level and in some geological areas of at least twice this. On the basis of all these considerations, the Commission recommends an annual limit on effective dose of 1 mSv. Averaging over time is discussed in the next paragraph.

(192) In deriving restrictions on sources of public exposure, some allowance is made for variations in the environmental pathways to man, but there will always be the possibility of larger transient changes. There will also be variations in the effectiveness of control procedures applied at the source and the Commission recommends that the transient increases in dose resulting from such variations should be included in the doses subject to the dose limits. Doses due to major accidents are not subject to the dose limits because they can be dealt with only by intervention. Since the detriment is a function of the accumulation of dose over many years, it would be unduly restrictive to require the controls to be related rigidly to annual dose limits. Some flexibility in the limits is desirable. The Commission's previous recommendations provided for a principal limit on the annual effective dose, with a subsidiary limit on the effective dose in some years, provided that the average effective dose over a lifetime did not exceed the principal limit. This recommendation is still sound in principle, but the Commission has concluded that the very long averaging period in the subsidiary limit gives excessive flexibility. It now recommends that the limit for public exposure should be expressed as an effective dose of 1 mSv in a year. However, in special circumstances, a higher value of effective dose could be allowed in a single year, provided that the average over 5 years does not exceed 1 mSv per year. Because this represents only a slight change from the previous recommendation, the Commission recommends that the 5-year period should be applied retrospectively when the new recommendation is being implemented. For this purpose, values of effective dose may be added to earlier values of effective dose equivalent. It is implicit in this limit that the constraints for the optimisation of protection in the design of new installations should be smaller than 1 mSv in a year.

(193) In selecting the limit on effective dose, the Commission has sought a value that would be only just short of unacceptable for continued exposure as the result of deliberate practices the use of which is a matter of choice. This does not imply that higher doses from other sources, such as radon in dwellings, should be regarded as unacceptable. The existence of these sources may be undesirable, but it is not a matter of choice. The doses can be controlled only by intervention, which will also have undesirable features.

(194) Limits are also needed for the lens of the eye and localised areas of skin since these tissues will not necessarily be protected against deterministic effects by the limit on effective dose. Because the total period of exposure may be nearly twice as long as for occupational exposure, and because the exposed individuals may show a wider range of sensitivity than the more limited population of workers, the recommended annual limits (non-occupational) for the equivalent dose in these tissues are lower than those for workers. The Commission has adopted an arbitrary reduction factor of 10, leading to annual limits of 15 mSv for the lens and 50 mSv averaged over any 1 cm² area of skin, regardless of the area exposed. The recommended limits are summarised in Table 6.

Table 6. Recommended dose limits[1]

Application	Dose limit Occupational	Public
Effective dose	20 mSv per year, averaged over defined periods of 5 years[2]	1 mSv in a year[3]
Annual equivalent dose in		
the lens of the eye	150 mSv	15 mSv
the skin[4]	500 mSv	50 mSv
the hands and feet	500 mSv	—

[1] The limits apply to the sum of the relevant doses from external exposure in the specified period and the 50-year committed dose (to age 70 years for children) from intakes in the same period (see paragraph 143).

[2] With the further provision that the effective dose should not exceed 50 mSv in any single year. Additional restrictions apply to the occupational exposure of pregnant women, which is discussed in Section 5.3.3.

[3] In special circumstances, a higher value of effective dose could be allowed in a single year, provided that the average over 5 years does not exceed 1 mSv per year.

[4] The limitation on the effective dose provides sufficient protection for the skin against stochastic effects. An additional limit is needed for localised exposures in order to prevent deterministic effects (see paragraphs 173 and 194).

5.6. Potential Exposures

(195) The initial treatment of potential exposures should form part of the system of protection applied to practices, but it should be recognised that the exposures, if they occur, may lead to intervention. At this stage, there should be two objectives, prevention and mitigation. Prevention is the reduction of the probability of the sequences of events that may cause or increase radiation exposures. It involves maintaining the reliability of all the operating and safety systems and of the associated working procedures. Mitigation is the limitation and reduction of the exposures if any of these sequences do occur. It involves the use of engineered safety features and operational procedures to control each sequence of events with the aim of limiting its consequences, should it occur. The arrangements for mitigation should not be restricted to plans for intervention. A great deal can be accomplished at the stages of design and operation to reduce the consequences of accident sequences so that intervention may not become necessary. It is difficult to compare, and to combine, the benefit of a reduction in probability (prevention) with that of a reduction in dose (mitigation) because a reduction in probability by a factor is not usually seen as equivalent to a reduction in dose by the same factor.

(196) In order to maintain a strict coherence in the treatment of actual and potential exposures, it would be necessary to extend the concept of detriment to include the probability of occurrence of the situation giving rise to the detriment. Techniques for achieving this are still being developed. Meanwhile, emphasis has to be placed on one part of the detriment, the probability of an attributable death. It must also be recognised that the uncertainties in estimating the probability of occurrence will usually be much greater than the uncertainties in estimating the probability of the consequences should the dose occur.

(197) The simplest way of dealing with the potential exposure of individuals is to consider the overall (*a priori*) individual probability of attributable death from cancer, rather than the effective dose, as the quantity to be used in the system of protection. For this purpose, the probability is defined as the product of the probability of incurring the dose and the lifetime conditional probability of attributable death from the dose if it were to have been incurred. A restriction corresponding to a dose limit can then be expressed in the form of a risk limit, i.e. a limit on the fatality probability. (See Section 5.6.3.) If the risk limit is derived from the probability of death attributable to exposure at the relevant dose limit, a corresponding level of protection will also be provided against non-fatal cancer and against deterministic effects.

(198) This use of the overall individual radiation risk is an adequate starting point for use in the system of protection, but it is not sufficient. This is because the situation will change if the event giving rise to the potential exposures actually occurs. At low probabilities of the potential event, an overall individual risk limit might imply doses when the event occurs that would be large enough to call for intervention or might result in deterministic effects. These undesirable outcomes should be borne in mind at the planning stage. They may call for lower risk constraints (analogous to dose constraints) than would be needed for high probability, low dose situations. When assessing the individual risk, it should be remembered that the conditional probability of deleterious effects if a dose is, in fact, incurred may be higher than the nominal probability because the doses and dose rates may be higher than those for which the nominal probability coefficients have been selected and because deterministic effects may become important at these higher doses.

(199) The specification of collective detriment from potential exposures is difficult and controversial, even if the consideration of detriment is limited to attributable deaths. It is not appropriate to depend on the use of the product of the probability of an event and the number of attributable deaths should it occur—the expectation value of the number of deaths—because this conceals the fact that the outcome will be either no consequences if the event does not occur, or the full consequences if it does. It also involves an implicit assumption of reciprocity between reductions in probability and reductions in the scale of consequences: i.e. the assumption that a frequent event with small consequences and a rare event with large consequences are equally detrimental if the expectation values of the consequences are the same.

(200) A more comprehensive approach to the collective detriment from potential exposures is that of multi-attribute analysis. Each characteristic (attribute) of the available options has to be identified and quantified. It is then given a weighting factor judged to represent its importance. The weighted attributes can then be aggregated to provide a figure of merit or compared individually with the weighted attributes in other options. Either method leads to a quantitative, or semi-quantitative, basis for choice between options.

(201) Meanwhile, a simpler approach is possible for both individual and collective

exposures if the doses will be small even if the event occurs. If the doses, should they occur, will not be in excess of dose limits, it is adequate to use the product of the expected dose and its probability of occurrence as if this were a dose that is certain to occur. The conventional procedures of justification and optimisation can then be applied.

5.6.1. Justification of a practice

(202) If sufficient information is available, the detriment associated with a proposed practice in the assessment of the justification of the practice should include that from the potential exposures. In practice, it may well be that the estimation of the detriment from potential exposures will be improved by operating experience obtained after the introduction of the practice. This will require a re-evaluation of the justification of the practice.

5.6.2. The optimisation of protection

(203) If the options for applying the system of protection to potential exposures do not alter the other exposures resulting from the practice, the potential detriment can be used in the procedures of optimisation without further complications. Sometimes, however, the two sets of exposure are interdependent and the optimisation of protection must then be carried out for both types of exposure together. (See Section 5.7.) In either case, the procedure must be constrained by an individual risk limit or, more probably, by source-related and sequence-related individual risk constraints.

5.6.3. Individual risk limits and constraints

(204) Although a risk limit can be defined by analogy with the dose limit, it will have a very different character. The probability of events leading to potential exposures cannot be determined by observation. They are the result of some form of probabilistic safety assessment. These assessments commonly provide estimates of the probability of defined accident sequences.

(205) The total probability from all possible sequences can be obtained only from a further stage of forecasting. It is therefore more useful to define a series of risk constraints applicable to the attributable probability of death, defined as the product of the probability of receiving a dose as the result of a precisely defined sequence and the lifetime conditional probability of attributable death from the dose if it were to have been received. Taken alone, these constraints will not be adequate because an individual will be at risk from more than one sequence. Unless there is one dominating sequence, there will also be a need for a risk limit, despite the difficulty of assessing the total risk to which the limit should apply. The Commission does not yet recommend an annual risk limit for individuals.

(206) There is also the possibility of potential doses in medical exposures. Errors in dosimetry and equipment failures have given rise to injurious, and sometimes fatal, doses to patients. The Commission does not recommend any specific value for risk constraints in this context.

5.7. Interactive Situations

(207) The bulk of the individual and collective doses often results from a single type of exposure. However, there are some cases where there is a significant contribution from several types of exposure.

(208) The first example is that of an interaction between public and occupational exposure. If the public exposure is due to the release of waste to the environment, a reduction in that exposure may result in increased occupational exposure due to the additional waste processing and storage. The simplest approach to the optimisation of protection is then to use the combined collective effective dose from the two forms of exposure. However, it has sometimes been considered that the detriment due to public exposure should be treated differently from that due to occupational exposure. This is not a view to which the Commission subscribes. The Commission recommends that the sum of the effective doses from each type of exposure from a given source should be used in the optimisation procedures. If the two components were thought to have different weightings, they could be used separately in a multi-attribute analysis.

(209) The second example is the interaction between potential exposure and occupational or public exposure. The mechanical inspection of plant may reduce the probability of failures but only at the expense of additional occupational exposure, and the reduction of public exposure by the increased storage of waste may cause increased potential occupational and public exposures. This form of interaction can be dealt with only by the methods of multi-attribute analysis.

6. THE SYSTEM OF PROTECTION IN INTERVENTION

Chapter 6 deals with situations where the sources of exposure and the exposure pathways are already present and the only type of action available is intervention. The chapter deals mainly with intervention applying to public exposure, including intervention following accidents, but includes some material on occupational exposure in emergencies. The practical application of these recommendations for intervention are discussed in Chapter 7.

(210) Before a programme of intervention is initiated, it should be demonstrated that the proposed intervention will be justified, i.e. do more good than harm, and that the form, scale, and duration of the intervention have been chosen so as to optimise the protection. As explained in Section 4.4 the Commission recommends against the use of dose limits for deciding on the need for, or scope of, intervention.

6.1. The Basis of Intervention in Public Exposure

(211) In judging the benefits and detriments of intervention aimed at reducing public exposure, the comparison should, in the first place, be made for those at risk, but there will also be an impact on the rest of society and the judgements will have to be wide enough to cover these impacts too.

(212) As indicated in Section 4.4, the processes of justification and optimisation both apply to the protective action, so it is necessary to consider them together when reaching a decision. Justification is the process of deciding that the disadvantages of each component of intervention, i.e. of each protective action, are more than offset by the reductions in the dose likely to be achieved. Optimisation is the process of deciding on the method, scale and duration of the action so as to obtain the maximum net benefit. The duration of countermeasures influences the averted dose and therefore the provisional

decision about the withdrawal of the countermeasures should be taken as part of the process of optimisation. In simple terms, the difference between the disadvantages and the benefits, expressed in the same terms, e.g. costs, including social costs with an allowance for anxiety, should be positive for each protective action adopted and should be maximised by settling the details of that action.

(213) The cost of intervention is not just the monetary cost. Some protective or remedial actions may involve non-radiological risks or serious social impacts. For example, the short-term removal of people from their homes is not very expensive, but it may cause the temporary separation of members of a family and result in considerable anxiety. Prolonged evacuation and permanent relocation are expensive and have sometimes been found to be highly traumatic.

(214) It follows from the above paragraphs that it is not possible to define quantitative intervention levels for rigid application in all circumstances. Nevertheless, because some kinds of action may be needed urgently, it is useful to have guidance prepared in advance for use following accidents and emergencies.

6.2. Situations in which Remedial Action may be Needed

(215) Many situations in which intervention is being considered are of long standing and do not call for urgent action. Others, resulting from accidents, may cause serious exposures unless immediate action can be taken. They may also cause long-term problems. The long-standing situations are dealt with in this section and the immediate problems of accidents in Section 6.3.

6.2.1. *Radon in dwellings*

(216) Radon in dwellings needs special attention because both the individual and the collective doses from radon are higher than those from almost any other source. In many countries, there are some individual doses substantially higher than those that would be permitted in occupational exposure. If improvements are needed, they have to be achieved by intervention involving modifications to the dwellings or to the behaviour of the occupants.

(217) In *Publication 39* (1984), the Commission recommended the use of action levels to help in deciding when to require or advise remedial action in existing dwellings. The choice of an action level is complex, depending not only on the level of exposure, but also on the likely scale of action, which has economic implications for the community and for individuals. For owner-occupied dwellings, general guidance may be adequate, leaving the final decision to be made by the occupier, on behalf of all the occupants, but in countries with substantial numbers of rented dwellings, it may be desirable to establish firm national action levels, at least for rented properties. In such cases, the best choice of an action level may well be that level which defines a significant, but not unmanageable, number of houses in need of remedial work. It is then not to be expected that the same action level will be appropriate in all countries.

(218) The problem of new dwellings has some similarity to that of existing dwellings because the concentration of radon cannot be determined with confidence until the dwelling has been completed and occupied for a year or so. It is then an existing dwelling. It is therefore dealt with here, rather than in Chapter 5. Guides or codes for the construction of new dwellings in selected areas can be established so that it is highly probable that they will result in exposures in these dwellings below some chosen reference level. The choice of this level may cause marked changes in conventional building practices and this

might have unforeseen effects on structures or living conditions. The Commission therefore wishes to proceed cautiously. It has initiated a further review of current experience with a view to issuing revised recommendations in due course. Meanwhile the guidance in *Publication 39* (1984) should still be used.

6.2.2. *Radioactive residues from previous events*

(219) The most common causes of residues are the burial of long-lived materials from early operations such as mining and luminising with radium compounds. The use of mining spoil as a land-fill material, followed by the construction of dwelling houses, has caused substantial problems. Buildings used for radium work have subsequently been put to other purposes, with the radium being discovered only years later. There have been several accidents in which long-lived radioactive materials have been dispersed in residential and agricultural areas. The necessary remedial actions vary greatly in complexity and scale and may themselves give rise to problems of occupational exposure and waste disposal. These should be dealt with in accordance with the Commission's recommendations for practices. The need for and extent of remedial action has to be judged by comparing the benefit of the reductions in dose with the detriment of the remedial work, including that due to the doses incurred in the remedial work. No general solutions are available, but the methods recommended for the optimisation of protection can be used to give guidance in each individual case.

6.3. Accidents and Emergencies

6.3.1. *Intervention affecting the public*

(220) The first step in deciding on the intervention likely to be needed after an accident is to define the type of all the likely protective actions and to consider the costs and the expected reductions in individual and collective doses as functions of the scale and duration of each. A substantial amount of preliminary work on economic and environmental models and on accident forecasting is needed for these assessments.

(221) Because the initial introduction of protective actions on any scale, however small, involves significant costs, it may well be that small-scale, short-duration, intervention is costly without being effective. As the scale and duration are increased, the effectiveness initially increases without a marked increase in costs. Eventually, further increases will fail to achieve increased benefits comparable with their costs and the net benefit again begins to fall. There is then a range of values of the possible intervention level of individual dose averted, within which there is an optimum level. If the net benefit at that optimum is positive, intervention of the defined type, scale and duration will be justified. The initial planning for emergencies should include the choice of intervention levels of dose averted, or a limited range of such intervention levels, that are likely to lead to intervention that is justified and reasonably well optimised.

(222) The benefit of a particular protective action within a programme of intervention should be judged on the basis of the reduction in dose achieved or expected by that specific protective action, the dose averted. Thus each protective action has to be considered on its own merits. For example, decisions about the control of individual foodstuffs are independent of decisions about other foodstuffs and of decisions about sheltering or evacuation. In addition, however, the doses that would be incurred via all the relevant pathways of exposure, some subject to protective actions and some not, should be assessed. If the total dose in some individuals is so high as to be unacceptable even in an emergency, the feasibility of additional protective actions influencing the

major contributions to the total dose should be urgently reviewed. Doses causing serious deterministic effects or a high probability of stochastic effects would call for such a review. For this purpose, an intervention level of dose received by all pathways should be chosen at the planning stage.

(223) The Commission has set out the general principles for planning intervention after an accident and included quantitative guidance on intervention levels in *Publication 40* (1984). This guidance was confined to short and medium term action. The Commission plans to issue further guidance covering the whole subject.

6.3.2. *The limitation of occupational exposure in emergencies*

(224) Occupational exposures directly due to an accident can be limited only by the design of the plant and its protective features and by the provision of emergency procedures. Ideally, the aim should be to keep the doses within those permitted in normal conditions, but, while this is usually possible, it may not always be so in serious accidents.

(225) In addition to the exposures resulting directly from the accident, there will be exposures of emergency teams during emergency and remedial action. Even in serious accidents, these can be limited by operational controls. The doses incurred are likely to be higher than in normal situations and should be treated separately from any normal doses. Emergencies involving significant exposures of emergency teams are rare, so some relaxation of the controls for normal situations can be permitted in serious accidents without lowering the long-term level of protection. This relaxation should not permit the exposures in the control of the accident and in the immediate and urgent remedial work to give effective doses of more than about 0.5 Sv except for life-saving actions, which can rarely be limited by dosimetric assessments. The equivalent dose to skin should not be allowed to exceed about 5 Sv, again except for life saving. Once the emergency is under control, remedial work should be treated as part of the occupational exposure incurred in a practice.

7. IMPLEMENTATION OF THE COMMISSION'S RECOMMENDATIONS

Chapter 7 emphasises the importance of the operational level of radiological protection and shows how this should be developed from the requirements of regulatory agencies and the recommendations of the Commission. It gives advice on the measurement of doses (monitoring) and on possible bases for exemption from regulatory requirements. It deals with both practices and intervention.

(226) This chapter is concerned principally with organisational features that may help in the implementation of the Commission's recommendations. Although the organisational structures will differ from country to country, and the chapter is therefore intended to be illustrative, the Commission hopes that it will provide useful guidance to managements and regulatory agencies.

(227) In the implementation of the Commission's recommendations, the main practical responsibilities fall on the designers and operators of equipment and installations, who obtain their guidance partly from professional advisors and publications such as those of the Commission and international organisations, and partly from regulatory and advisory bodies. Governments should establish a framework of regulatory and advisory

functions aimed at helping the operating managements to meet their responsibilities and at ensuring that a suitable standard of protection is maintained. This framework should also make provision for any necessary central services, including those for intervention, and for links to regional and international organisations in both normal and emergency situations.

(228) The organisational structures used in the control of practices should, as far as possible, also be used to deal with intervention, although they will have to be modified and extended in some respects. This will help to maintain consistency and will avoid too much dependency on lines of demarcation. Planning for intervention in the event of emergences should be an integral part of normal operating procedures. Any changes in responsibility, e.g. from the usual line of command to an emergency controller, should be planned in advance. The hand-over should be a formal procedure. More details are given in Section 7.7. When there is no operating management, e.g. for radon in dwellings, intervention should become the responsibility of the regulatory agency or of some other clearly defined body.

(229) The Commission's recommendations have been set out as a sequence of concepts, starting with the primary aims and broadening out to cover more detailed aspects. This structure has been followed in this chapter, which shows how the responsibilities of the various bodies are interrelated. To do this it is necessary to establish a logical sequence of stages, as follows:

Allocation of responsibility
Basic recommendations of the Commission
Requirements of regulatory agencies
Management requirements
Validation of performance

To a large extent, these stages are the same for all types of exposure. However, when intervention is required, there may not always be a relevant operating management available and the regulatory agency, or some other designated body, will have to accept some of the responsibilities usually carried by the operating management.

7.1. Responsibility and Authority

(230) In radiological protection, as in other matters concerning health and safety, it is often convenient to distinguish between responsibility and authority. The first stage of **responsibility** is the duty to establish objectives, to provide the measures needed to achieve those objectives, and to ensure that these measures are properly carried out. This is essentially a prospective concept. Those bearing responsibility should then have the **authority** to commit the resources needed to meet their responsibilities. There is also a retrospective component of responsibility, sometimes called **accountability**, that requires a continuing review of performance to be made so that failures can be identified and steps taken to prevent recurrence. Accountability implies the need to establish a programme of verification to determine how effectively the original objectives are being achieved.

(231) The primary responsibility for achieving and maintaining a satisfactory control of radiation exposures rests squarely on the management bodies of the institutions conducting the operations giving rise to the exposures. When equipment or plant is designed and supplied by other institutions, they, in turn, have a responsibility to see that the items supplied will be satisfactory, if used as intended. Governments have the

responsibility to set up regulatory agencies, which then have the responsibility for providing a regulatory, and often also an advisory, framework to emphasise the responsibilities of the management bodies while, at the same time, setting and enforcing overall standards of protection. They may also have to take direct responsibility when, as with exposures to many natural sources, there is no relevant management body.

(232) In all organisations, the responsibilities and the associated authority are delegated to an extent depending on the complexity of the duties involved. The working of this delegation should be examined regularly. There should be a clear line of accountability running right to the top of each organisation. The delegation of responsibilities does not detract from that accountability. There is also an interaction between the various kinds of organisation. Advisory and regulatory agencies should be held accountable for the advice they give and any requirements they impose. The imposition of requirements expressed in general terms and the acceptance of advice do not reduce the responsibility, or the accountability, of the operating organisations. This is also true of prescriptive requirements expressed in terms of objectives or limits. Prescriptive requirements concerning the conduct of operations do, however, result in some de facto transfer of responsibility and accountability from the operator to the regulator. The use of such requirements can be very effective, especially where the operating management lacks detailed experience, but such use always needs to be carefully justified.

(233) Requirements, operating instructions, regulatory approvals and licences and other administrative devices are not, of themselves, enough to achieve an appropriate standard of radiological protection. Everyone in an undertaking, from the individual workers and their representatives to the senior management, should regard protection and accident prevention as integral parts of their every-day functions. Success and failure in these areas are at least as important as they are in the primary function of the undertaking.

7.2. The Recommendations of the Commission

(234) As indicated in Section 1.3, the recommendations of the Commission are intended, *inter alia*, to provide a useful basis from which to derive the necessary regulatory requirements. Subject to any mandatory requirements of the regulatory agencies, the recommendations also provide guidance to the operating managements. The widespread adoption of the recommendations has the advantage of giving a consistency of aims and standards across a wide range of countries. It also helps to provide an appropriate degree of uniformity of procedures. To assist in this process, the Commission has tried to make clear the reasons for its recommendations and has deliberately included some flexibility, so that consistency can be obtained without rigidity.

(235) Widespread acceptance of the quantities discussed in Chapter 2 and of the proposed values of the nominal probability coefficient, the radiation weighting factors, w_R, and the tissue weighting factors, w_T, will greatly simplify world-wide comparisons of doses and practices and will help in the development of engineering standards for instrument design and performance.

7.3. Regulatory Requirements

(236) The form of regulatory agencies, their requirements, and their methods of operating differ widely. Regulatory provisions are not an alternative to management

requirements: they are better seen as a bridge between the recommendations of the Commission and the management requirements. In some respects they should go further. In particular, a large part of the duty of assessing the justification of a practice should rest on the regulatory agency or on the government upon which it depends. Provisions may be needed to prohibit practices not regarded as being justified. The regulatory provisions should also set a broad and adequate standard of protection for application to the practices that are regarded as justified.

(237) One important national and international need is to provide adequate resources for the education and training of future professional and technical staff in radiological protection. These resources cannot be provided by the regulatory agencies alone.

7.3.1. *The regulation of practices*

(238) One feature of the regulation of practices is the use of source-related con- straints to be applied to the optimisation of protection. It will avoid confusion if it is made clear that these regulatory constraints are not the same as prescriptive regulatory limits. Limits prescribed by regulatory agencies and restrictions applied by managements to specific operations as part of the day-to-day control of exposures are not constraints in the sense used here. In general, they should be established on the basis of the results of optimisation. However, some regulatory agencies use prescribed limits as a form of regulatory constraint, requiring the operating management to achieve further reductions based on optimisation. Prescriptive limits may apply not only to dose but also to any features that are under the direct control of the operating management, such as releases to the environment. The purpose of prescriptive limits should be clarified when they are being set. In any event, they should never be regarded as an alternative to the process of optimising protection. It is not satisfactory to set design or operational limits or targets as an arbitrary fraction of the dose limit, regardless of the particular nature of the plant and the operations.

(239) A high proportion of operations can be conducted in such a way that the standard of protection is set by the process of constrained optimisation and not by the dose limits. Mandatory dose constraints, applicable to selected classes of operation, then provide a useful regulatory tool. Alternatively, the regulatory agency might establish investigation levels for classes of operation. Exceeding an investigation level would require an investigation to be made of the optimisation programme of the operator or designer.

(240) Occasionally, an individual is seen to be consistently exposed at a high level, close to the individual dose limit, so that the accumulated effective dose may be approaching an unacceptable level. Special attention should then be given to the justifi- cation of the practice and the optimisation of protection. This may lead to the imposition of a special prescriptive limit aimed at forcing an improvement, or to the use of an investigation level requiring a formal review of the procedures for optimising protection.

(241) The regulatory agencies should be particularly concerned with public exposures because of the possibility of individuals' being exposed to more than one source. This makes it particularly important to identify lines of responsibility and to establish clearly to which sources the regulatory provisions apply.

(242) The regulatory provisions may be of a general nature, or they may be related directly to one installation or to a class of installations. In each case, the agency will have to consider both the source-related approach, to ensure the proper optimisation of protection, including the selection of source-related dose constraints, and the individual-

related approach to ensure the adequate protection of individuals in relation to all the relevant sources. If the primary source is not under the jurisdiction of the agency, e.g. when radioactive material is released to a river upstream of the agency's area, it may be useful to consider assessments and controls to be related to a particular sector of the environment. Control cannot then be applied at the source, so that doses can be limited, if at all, only by some form of intervention. It will usually be better to achieve control of the source by inter-state, or inter-agency, collaboration.

(243) The objectives, and to some extent the methods, of regulatory agencies may sometimes be subject to formal international or regional requirements. Most of these are advisory, but some are mandatory, at least as far as objectives are concerned. There is also a range of international engineering standards, some of which have a bearing on radiological protection. The responsible international bodies also issue advisory documents. All these documents provide a valuable input to the process of achieving an appropriate level of protection.

7.3.2. *Regulation in the context of potential exposures*

(244) The first step in regulation in the context of potential exposures is that of establishing a duty on the operating management to conduct assessments of the expected frequency and possible consequences of events, such as accidents and major errors of design and operation, that might give rise to doses substantially higher than those in normal conditions. Account should be taken of a wide range of initiating causes, including those outside the operator's control, e.g. floods and storms. The operator should be required to include a review of the procedures necessary to deal with the events, should they occur. These assessments will necessarily be based on identified sequences of events: it will rarely be possible to ensure that all such sequences have been identified. The possible existence of rare unidentified sequences makes it impossible to justify assessments leading to very low values of the overall probability of accidents.

(245) The second stage is that of regulatory review. Depending on the likely scale of the problems posed by the events giving rise to potential exposures, the regulatory agency should establish a procedure for reviewing the operators' assessments. In most cases, this need be no more than the conventional level of testing for compliance with any regulatory requirement. In the few installations where the consequences of an accident might be severe, the procedure may involve a detailed review of the whole assessment, possibly linked to a system of prior approval or licensing. The use of risk constraints related to individual sequences should be considered. These may make it unnecessary to establish overall risk limits, which are difficult to select and even more difficult to enforce.

(246) Compliance with risk limits and constraints has to be judged from the results of assessments of the quality of the design, operation and maintenance of the plant and equipment and the quality of the management arrangements. Relevant features include the performance and reliability of equipment and the quality of test procedures, operating instructions and training.

7.4. Management Requirements

(247) The first, and in many ways the most important, of the practical steps in implementing the Commission's recommendations is the establishment of a safety-based attitude in everyone concerned with all the operations from design to decommissioning.

This can only be achieved by a substantial commitment to training and a recognition that safety is a personal responsibility and is of major concern to the top management. Close links between the management and the representatives of the workforce have a major role to play.

(248) This attitude to safety should be reinforced by the creation of a formal management structure for dealing with radiological protection, including the optimisation of protection, and by the issuing of clear operating instructions. These should take account of any requirements applied to the design of the plant and equipment and of the installation as a whole, and should cover subsidiary operations such as inspection and maintenance. The details of the management structure and of the operating instructions will depend on the form and scale of the operating organisation, but their importance should be recognised even in small or informal organisations. From the point of view of the Commission, it is convenient to consider design requirements and operating instructions as parts of a unified system, to be called the management requirements, even though the two parts may be laid down by different components of the management organisation.

(249) The aims of the management requirements should be to set out the practical basis for protecting all concerned. The detailed techniques cover such aspects as the choice of radiation source or radioactive material, the use of shielding and distance to reduce radiation fields, the restriction of the time spent in the proximity of sources, and the use of containment, usually in several stages, to limit the spread of radioactive materials into workplaces and the public environment. Attention should also be given to the layout of plant and equipment. In addition, the techniques for dealing with potential exposures include safety analysis to identify possible causes of accidents and the methods available to reduce their likelihood and severity, followed by the assessment of the reliability of all the principal systems affecting the probability of accidents. These systems include the plant and equipment, any software used in the equipment or in the operations, the operating and maintenance procedures, and the performance of the human operators. Much of the responsibility for these analyses should fall on the designer, but part of it should rest on the operating management. There should be plans for dealing with accidents should they occur. These plans should be subject to periodic review. All these reviews and assessments should lead to the preparation of written management requirements.

(250) The management requirements should be expressed in clear and unambiguous terms and they should be eminently practical. They will stem, in part, from the requirements of regulatory agencies (see Section 7.3), but they should also draw on the recommendations of the Commission, manuals of good practice, and engineering standards. The task of preparing and implementing management requirements is onerous, but it plays an important part in achieving the correct balance between the protection measures and the effective conduct of the operations.

7.4.1. *The classification of workplaces and working conditions*

(251) One of the most important functions of management requirements is that of maintaining control over the sources of exposure and over the workers who are occupationally exposed. It is usually easy to specify the sources of occupational exposure. They are the artificial radioactive materials and the electrical generators of radiation used in the workplace, together with the natural sources specified in Section 5.1.1. The specification has to be applied with common-sense because artificial radionuclides are

present in trace amounts in most materials. The control of sources is helped by requiring that the workplaces containing them be formally designated. The Commission uses two such designations—controlled areas and supervised areas.

(252) A controlled area is one in which normal working conditions, including the possible occurrence of minor mishaps, require the workers to follow well-established procedures and practices aimed specifically at controlling radiation exposures. A supervised area is one in which the working conditions are kept under review but special procedures are not normally needed. The definitions are best based on operational experience and judgement. Account should be taken both of the expected levels of exposure and of the likely variations in these exposures. In areas where there is no problem of contamination by unsealed radioactive materials, designated areas may sometimes be defined in terms of the dose rates at the boundary. The aim should be to ensure that anyone outside the designated areas will not need to be regarded as occupationally exposed. The dose limits recommended by the Commission are intended to apply to all workers, but the use of designated areas should enable the actual doses received outside the designated areas to be kept below the dose limits for public exposure. The dividing line between controlled areas and supervised areas, if the latter are used, has commonly been set with the aim of ensuring that the doses to workers in the supervised areas can confidently be predicted to be less than 3/10 of the occupational dose limits. The Commission now regards this definition as being too arbitrary and recommends that the designation of controlled and supervised areas should be decided either at the design stage or locally by the operating management on the basis of operational experience and judgement. This judgement has to take account of the expected level and the likely variations of the doses and intakes, and the potential for accidents.

(253) In previous recommendations, the Commission has defined two types of working conditions based on the expected level of individual annual dose. This was originally intended to help in the choice of workers to be subject to individual monitoring and special medical surveillance. In recent years, it has become apparent that neither of these decisions is best linked to a crude classification of working conditions based on expected dose and the Commission no longer recommends such a classification. The design of monitoring programmes is discussed in Section 7.5.1 and medical surveillance in Section 7.4.4.

7.4.2. *Operational guides*

(254) Generalised exhortations to keep risks low are implicit in radiological protection. They should be supplemented by specific statements that the designers and the operators can use as guides. The operating management is responsible for establishing these guides, which should include an indication of the maximum levels of exposure that the management expects to occur in defined operations.

(255) These guides apply to both the designers and operators of plant and equipment, but they are not targets and are not sufficient. They provide only an envelope within which the designers and operators should work. In addition, there should be an obligation to consider the available options and to establish operational procedures based on more completely optimised levels of protection for the specific circumstances. These operational guides are becoming increasingly common and are to be welcomed, provided that they are soundly based. If operational guides are chosen to be the same for widely diverse operations, they are likely to be arbitrary and will not be consistent with the standards of protection recommended by the Commission.

(256) In principle, the operational guides should include material on the standard of

reliability needed to limit potential exposures. In practice, however, it is proving difficult to establish a sound basis for such material, sometimes known as "safety goals". It is therefore necessary to depend heavily on past experience, often codified in the form of engineering standards.

7.4.3. *Reference levels*

(257) It is often helpful in the management of operations to establish values of measured quantities above which some specified action or decision should be taken. These values are generally called reference levels. They include recording levels, above which a result should be recorded, lower values being ignored; investigation levels, above which the cause or the implications of the result should be examined; and intervention levels, above which some remedial action should be considered. The use of these levels can avoid unnecessary or unproductive work and can help in the effective deployment of resources. If recording levels are used, the fact that no unrecorded results exceeded the recording level should be made clear.

7.4.4. *Occupational services for protection and health*

(258) One common responsibility of the operating management is to provide access to occupational services dealing with protection and health. These may be in-house services or consultancy services brought in from outside. The protection service should provide specialist advice and arrange any necessary monitoring provisions, both inside and outside the installation. The head of the protection service should have direct access to the senior operating management. Most of this report has already been concerned with the provisions for protection. This section therefore concentrates on the provision of occupational health services.

(259) The principal role of the occupational health service is the same as it is in any occupation. Physicians supervising the health of a force of radiation workers need to be familiar with the tasks and working conditions of the workforce. They then have to decide on the fitness of each worker for the intended tasks. It is now very rare for the radiation component of the working environment to have any significant influence on that decision. Furthermore, this component should have no influence on the administrative conditions of service of those occupationally exposed.

(260) The supervising physician, sometimes supported by specialists, may also be required to counsel workers in three special categories. The first is women who are, or may become, pregnant. They should be advised to inform the physician as soon as they think they may be pregnant, so that the management can be advised to arrange for any necessary change of duties or special protective provisions.

(261) The second group comprises any individuals who have been exposed substantially in excess of the dose limits or may have been involved in potentially dangerous situations. Only in exceptional conditions will clinical tests or treatment be indicated. Nevertheless, depending on the potential for accidents, the physician should ensure that suitable arrangements for diagnostic tests and treatment can be provided at short notice if they should be required. One laboratory test to be considered in this context is the examination of lymphocytes for chromosome aberrations. This test can often give useful results and reassurance after suspected accidents. In-house provisions are rarely needed because there are laboratories in many countries to which blood samples can be sent.

(262) The third group comprises individual workers who are considering volunteering for deliberate exposures as part of biomedical research programmes. In well-designed

experiments, the doses will be small compared with those commonly incurred in occupational exposure and will be limited by dose constraints applied in the optimisation of protection. The supervising physician can provide reassurance and can exclude any volunteers expressing anxiety. Reference to a properly constituted ethics committee is needed to ensure that the research aims are proper and well defined and that the system for selecting volunteers is satisfactory.

(263) The supervising physician needs information about the working conditions and the exposures of individual workers. Some of this information will come from plant records, and some from the protection service. Some of the data will be transferred to, and then form part of, the individual's medical record. Such records are usually regarded as medically confidential. It is important not to let confidentiality compromise the availability of the original data to the management and to non-medical professionals involved in protection.

7.5. The Assessment of Doses

(264) The basis of the Commission's recommendations is the restriction of doses and of the probability of incurring doses. The measurement or assessment of doses is fundamental to the practice of radiological protection. Neither the equivalent dose in an organ nor the effective dose can be measured directly. Values of these quantities must be inferred with the aid of models, usually involving environmental, metabolic, and dosimetric components. Ideally, these models and the values chosen for their parameters should be realistic, so that the results they give can be described as "best estimates". Where practicable, estimates should be made of the uncertainties inherent in these results.

(265) In practice, realistic models are rarely available. If the purposes of the model includes the setting of limits or the subsequent testing for compliance with limits, and if realistic models are not available, it is appropriate to use models that are intended to give results that are not likely to underestimate the consequences of exposure, though without overestimating the consequences excessively. In the justification of a practice, the optimisation of protection, or the decision to use intervention following an accident, any errors of estimation are liable to cause misuse of resources. If the models are to be used solely for these purposes, they should therefore be chosen with the emphasis on realism.

7.5.1. Dosimetry in occupational exposure

(266) In occupational exposure, it is usually feasible to monitor the doses received by individuals. Often, however, there is no clear-cut line between workers closely involved with radiation sources and others who are exposed only casually, either because they are rarely present in the relevant locations or because they are remote and receive only trivial doses. To avoid a wasteful use of resources in monitoring and record keeping, it is necessary to identify groups of workers for whom individual monitoring is needed.

(267) The decision to provide individual monitoring for a group of workers depends on many factors. Some of these are technical and others are concerned more with industrial relations. The decision should be taken by the operating management, but should be subject to review by the regulatory agency. Three major technical factors should influence the decision; the expected level of dose or intake in relation to the relevant limits, the likely variations in the dose and intakes, and the complexity of the measurement and interpretation procedures comprising the monitoring programme. This

third factor results in an approach to the monitoring for external exposure that is different from that for intakes and the resulting committed effective dose. Individual monitoring for external radiation is fairly simple and does not require a heavy commitment of resources. It should be used for all those who are occupationally exposed, unless it is clear that their doses will be consistently low, or, as in the case of air crew, it is clear that the circumstances prevent the doses from exceeding an identified value. In addition to its primary function of providing information for the control of exposures, a programme of individual monitoring may be helpful in confirming the classification of workplaces and in detecting fluctuations in working conditions. It gives useful reassurance and may provide data of use in reviewing optimisation programmes.

(268) Individual monitoring for intakes of radioactive material is usually much more difficult, and should be used routinely only for workers who are employed in areas that are designated as controlled areas specifically in relation to the control of contamination and in which there are grounds for expecting significant intakes. Guidance on the type of work calling for individual monitoring is given in *Publication 35* (1982). Guidance on the interpretation of individual monitoring for intakes is given in *Publication 54* (1988).

(269) When calculating the annual limits on intake (ALIs), the Commission has previously used the 50-year committed effective dose. For workers with a working life from 18 to 65 years (a mean of about 40 years) and an expectation of living to 75 years, a value of 35 years would be more typical. However, the difference is small, even for long-lived, long retained, nuclides, and the Commission recommends the retention of the 50-year period for occupational exposure. (See Section 7.5.3 for Public Exposure.) In discussions with an individual worker of the possible health implications of his monitoring results, account should be taken of the actual age at intake. The intake can be directly related to the annual limit on intake more convincingly than the committed dose can be related to the annual dose limit so it will usually be more satisfactory to discuss estimated intakes rather than committed doses.

(270) The assessment of collective dose from occupational exposure is usually based on the recorded doses from individual monitoring programmes, but will often have to be supplemented by the use of data on low individual doses derived from models based on measurements in the workplace.

(271) In practice, it is usually possible without great difficulty to achieve an accuracy of about 10% at the 95% confidence level for measurements of radiation fields in good laboratory conditions. In the workplace, where the energy and orientation of the radiation field are rarely known, uncertainties by a factor of 1.5 will not be unusual in the estimation of annual doses from the external exposure of individual workers. In view of the other uncertainties, this factor is acceptable. It will rarely be possible to achieve the same standard of accuracy when estimating intakes and the associated committed equivalent and effective doses. Uncertainties by a factor of at least 3 may well have to be recognised and are acceptable. Further guidance is given in *Publication 54* (1988).

7.5.2. *Dosimetry in medical exposure*

(272) The assessment of doses in medical exposure, i.e. doses to patients, is of critical importance in radiotherapy and is dealt with by the International Commission on Radiation Units and Measurements. Frequent measurements on equipment should form an important part of the quality control programme. In diagnostic radiology, there is rarely a need for routine assessment of doses, but periodic measurements should be made to check the performance of equipment and to encourage the optimisation of

protection. In nuclear medicine, the administered activity should always be recorded and the doses, based on standard models, will then be readily available.

7.5.3. *Dosimetry in public exposure*

(273) Routine individual monitoring of persons subject to public exposure is not necessary in normal situations and is not recommended. Dose assessment is then dependent on models representing the pathways between the source and the exposed individuals, sometimes supplemented by environmental monitoring. This procedure cannot take full account of individual habits and characteristics. For comparisons with limits, the models should relate to real or postulated "critical groups". These groups are chosen to be representative of the individuals most highly exposed as a result of the source under review. They are required to be reasonably homogeneous with respect to the characteristics that influence their doses from that source. When this is achieved, any individual limits should be applied to the mean values for the critical group. The Commission has dealt with the selection of critical groups in *Publication 43* (1985).

(274) For public exposure, the integrating period for committed effective dose for children should be from the age of the intake to 70 years. For adults, the period should be 50 years. The Commission has provided age-specific relationships between intake and committed effective dose in *Publication 56* (1989).

(275) In public exposure, it is rare for the collective dose to be predominantly composed of doses in members of the critical group. Dose assessment for the purposes of justification of a practice or the optimisation of protection has to be based on more general models. For current situations, and those extending only into the near future, such models can sometimes be validated by selective measurements, for example on environmental materials or, more rarely, on individuals. For longer-term predictive models, which are often used to forecast doses over many centuries and over large areas, no direct validation is possible. However, techniques such as sensitivity and uncertainty analysis are useful in indicating the likely degree of error and make it possible to test any proposed choice of action against a range of predictive models.

7.6. Compliance with the Intended Standard of Protection

(276) All the organisations concerned with radiological protection should have a duty to verify their compliance with their own objectives and procedures. The operating management should establish a system for reviewing its organisational structure and its procedures, a function analogous to financial auditing. Regulatory agencies should conduct similar internal audits and should have the added duty of, and authority for, assessing both the level of protection achieved by operating managements and the degree of compliance with the regulatory provisions. All these verification procedures should include consideration of potential exposures by a verification of the safety provisions. Verification procedures should include a review of quality assurance programmes and some form of inspection. However, inspection is a form of sampling—it cannot cover all eventualities. It is best seen as a mechanism for persuading those inspected to put, and keep, their own houses in order.

7.6.1. *Record keeping*

(277) Any system of validation includes the keeping of records. The minimum requirements will usually be laid down by the regulatory agencies, but operating manage-

ments should consider the additional requirements for records for their own purposes. The type of record, the degree of detail, and the retention period should all be defined formally. A balance has to be struck between the complexity of the initial entry of data, which may compromise the accuracy or completeness, and the possible future use of the records. The value of most records decreases with time, as does the likelihood of their being needed. As a general guide, and subject to any regulatory requirements, records giving the results of assessments of individual doses should be retained for periods comparable with the expected lifetime of the individual; those giving supplementary information used in the interpretation of monitoring results, e.g. results of monitoring of the workplace, should be retained for a period long enough to keep them available for any likely re-assessment of the interpretation, a few years. The details and retention of personnel records should be in accordance with the normal practice of the employer. The details of releases of waste to the environment should be retained for at least 10 years, with summaries being kept for several decades.

7.7. Emergency Planning

(278) When an emergency that may affect the public is declared, there should usually be a shift in the placing of responsibilities. In many cases, there will be an operating management at the scene of the initiating event. The operating management will then be available to take initial control of the event itself, but this may not be regarded as appropriate if the event is outside, or extends beyond, the operator's premises. The wider responsibilities for emergency action will usually have to be carried by the regulatory agency, which will also have to decide who shall be responsible for implementing any action following its decisions.

(279) Accidents or operational misjudgements may call for urgent action. The responsibility for planning local emergency action should fall primarily on the operating management, if this can be identified in advance. More general, and especially national, planning should be the responsibility of the regulatory agency or other body designated by the Government. Local and national plans need to be closely co-ordinated and linked to other plans dealing with accidents not involving radiation. Links to regional and international plans should also be provided. Bilateral agreements with neighbouring states are often needed and are essential where major installations are located near national boundaries. The scale of the detailed plans for dealing with radiation accidents will be influenced by the degree of co-ordination with other plans and by the magnitude and expected frequency of accidents. The establishment, maintenance, and exercising of emergency plans require a substantial commitment of resources, so the choice of the scale of the plans has considerable practical implications.

(280) Experience has identified several key areas of difficulty in emergency planning. The first is the recognition that an accident has occurred and that emergency action is needed. This presents few difficulties if the accident is to major plant, but dangerous situations due to lost or misused radiographic sources have been very difficult to recognise. The second problem area is the rapid acquisition and interpretation of data. It is obvious that data have to be obtained in the area affected by the accident, but it is not always recognised that there will be a widespread demand for data to provide reassurance in unaffected areas. Thirdly, the interpreted data have to lead to decisions and actions, or to a convincing conclusion that no action is needed. The initial decisions will often have to made by someone on the spot, regardless of the formal chain of responsi-

bilities. This should be recognised in the plans, but provision should also be made for the more formal making of decisions on a longer timescale. The fourth problem area is communications. The demand for information has been consistently underestimated in the past. The communication system for the emergency organisation is not difficult to specify, but it is expensive to establish and maintain. Adequate communications with the public are very much more difficult to achieve. The provision of local instructions and advice in the event of an accident is fairly straightforward, once the content has been settled. It is much more difficult to disseminate reassurance to the much larger areas where no action is called for. Special provisions should be made in national plans.

(281) Because of these special features, there are many parts of emergency plans that are not in routine use. These have to be maintained in a state of readiness by regular exercises. Exercises are often regarded as wasteful of scarce resources, but they should be treated as a necessary part of emergency planning.

(282) It is necessary to initiate emergency procedures by some form of declaration of a state of emergency. This may be local, perhaps applying only to a single installation, or even to a single workplace, or it may be more widespread. Such a declaration has the additional function of establishing that the system of protection is now that relating to intervention. Provision also has to be made for the withdrawal of the state of emergency and of any countermeasures that have been applied.

(283) Although flexibility is a necessary feature of emergency plans, it is very valuable to include in the plans a set of intervention levels to provide an immediate basis for urgent decisions. These intervention levels should be established for the types of action likely to be needed and should be promulgated by, or on behalf of, the regulatory agency. As discussed in Chapter 6, the choice of intervention levels should be based on the dose averted by the proposed action. Since the dose that will be averted cannot easily be estimated in the period immediately after an accident, derived intervention levels should be established for quantities that can be measured or estimated at the time of use. The intervention levels should not be treated as limits, they are guides to action.

(284) To avoid unnecessary restrictions in international trade, especially in foodstuffs, it may be necessary, in this context, to apply derived intervention levels in a different way. They could then indicate a line of demarcation between freely permitted exports or imports and those that should be the subject of special decisions. Any restrictions applied to goods below the intervention levels, better called intervention exemption levels for this purpose, should be regarded as artificial barriers to trade. Trade in materials above an intervention exemption level should not automatically be prohibited, but such materials might be subject to temporary controls. Intervention exemption levels used in this way in international trade should not necessarily have the same quantitative values as the intervention levels used for initiating action in other circumstances.

7.8. Exclusion and Exemption from Regulatory Control

(285) In order to avoid excessive regulatory procedures, most regulatory systems include provisions for granting exemptions in cases where it is clear that a practice is justified, but where regulatory provisions are unnecessary. Provision may also be made for the complete exclusion of some situations from the scope of any regulatory instruments.

(286) The Commission believes that the exemption of sources is an important component of the regulatory functions. It notes that the International Atomic Energy

Agency and the Nuclear Energy Agency of OECD issue advice on this subject to their member states.

(287) There are two grounds for exempting a source or an environmental situation from regulatory control. One is that the source gives rise to small individual doses and small collective doses in both normal and accident conditions. The other is that no reasonable control procedures can achieve significant reductions in individual and collective doses.

(288) The basis for exemption on the grounds of trivial dose is much sought after, but very difficult to establish. Apart from the difficulty of deciding when an individual or a collective dose is small enough to be disregarded for regulatory purposes, there is a considerable difficulty in defining the source. For example, if the source is defined as a single smoke detector, both the individual and the collective doses from that source may well be trivial, but the individual may be exposed to many other sources. If the source is taken as smoke detectors in general, the individual doses will still be small, but the collective dose may be substantial. The underlying problem is that exemption is necessarily a source-related process, while the triviality of the dose is primarily individual-related.

(289) When the exempt source comprises a class of devices, it may not be appropriate to exempt the manufacture and large scale storage of the devices. The devices themselves can be made subject to the requirements of approved engineering standards, and their sale and use can then be exempted from all further regulatory requirements. When the use is so exempted, it is necessary also to be able to exempt the eventual disposal of the devices.

(290) The second basis for exemption calls for a study similar to that needed in the optimisation of protection. It provides a logical basis for exemption of sources that cannot be exempted solely on the grounds of trivial doses, but for which regulation on any reasonable scale will produce little or no improvement.

(291) Sources that are essentially uncontrollable, such as cosmic radiation at ground level and potassium-40 in the body, can best be dealt with by the process of exclusion from the scope of the regulatory instruments, rather than by an exemption provision forming part of the regulatory instruments.

(292) One other form of exemption is sometimes considered. Some sources give rise to widespread exposures involving only very small individual doses. It has been suggested that these sources could be exempted from regulatory concern and the small individual doses might be excluded from the calculation of collective dose. In effect, it is argued that the resulting risks to individuals are so insignificant that they can be ignored even if there are many exposed individuals. In the context of waste management, this approach tends to ignore large collective doses delivered at long ranges, often in other countries. This method of exemption is sometimes the result of an implicit form of optimisation of protection. If the doses are individually small and the sources are widespread, it may well be impossible to reduce the doses further with any reasonable deployment of resources. It is unlikely, however, that this argument would lead to a single value of dose for exemption purposes.

(293) The Commission recognises that this method of exemption, i.e. ignoring the collective dose if the individual doses are all very small, is in use, not always explicitly, and that it often leads to conclusions that are broadly consistent with those that would result from the application of the Commission's system of protection. Nevertheless, this consistency is not always achieved and the Commission does not recommend the use of

this technique. The extent to which small individual doses should be included in the estimation of collective doses for the purposes of optimisation depends on the extent to which the contribution from these doses influences the choice between the options under review. Further guidance is given in *Publication 55* (1989).

SUMMARY OF RECOMMENDATIONS

This summary contains the principal recommendations and new concepts in the 1990 Recommendations of the Commission. Explanatory material is omitted. The order of the summary follows that of the Main Text of the recommendations.

Introduction

(S1) The Recommendations are intended to be of help to regulatory and advisory agencies and to management bodies and their professional staff. They deal only with ionising radiation and with the protection of man. The Commission emphasises that ionising radiation needs to be treated with care rather than fear and that its risks should be kept in perspective with other risks. Radiological protection cannot be conducted on the basis of scientific considerations alone. All those concerned have to make value judgements about the relative importance of different kinds of risk and about the balancing of risks and benefits.

Quantities Used in Radiological Protection

(S2) The Commission uses macroscopic dosimetric quantities while recognising that microdosimetric quantities based on the statistical distribution of events in a small volume of material may eventually be more appropriate. The principal dosimetric quantities in radiological protection are the mean absorbed dose in a tissue or organ, D_T, the energy absorbed per unit mass; the equivalent dose in a tissue or organ, H_T, formed by weighting the absorbed dose by the radiation weighting factor, w_R; and the effective dose, E, formed by weighting the equivalent dose by the tissue weighting factor, w_T, and summing over the tissues. The time integral of the effective-dose rate following an intake of a radionuclide is called the committed effective dose, $E(\tau)$, where τ is the integration time (in years) following the intake. The unit of absorbed dose is the gray (Gy), and the unit of both equivalent and effective dose is the sievert (Sv). The values of the radiation and tissue weighting factors are given in Tables S-1 and S-2.

(S3) Another useful quantity is the collective effective dose, which is the product of the mean effective dose in a group and the number of individuals in that group. With some reservations, it can be thought of as representing the total consequences of the exposure of a population or group.

(S4) The Commission uses "dose" as a generic term that can apply to any of the relevant dosimetric quantities. The Commission also uses the term "exposure" in a generic sense to mean the process of being exposed to radiation or radioactive material. The significance of an exposure in this sense is determined by the resulting doses.

Biological Aspects of Radiological Protection

(S5) Ionising radiation causes both deterministic and stochastic effects in irradiated tissue. Radiological protection aims at avoiding deterministic effects by setting dose limits below their thresholds. Stochastic effects are believed to occur, albeit with low frequency, even at the lowest doses and therefore have been taken into account at all doses.

Table S-1. Radiation weighting factors[1]

Type and energy range[2]	Radiation weighting factor, w_R
Photons, all energies	1
Electrons and muons, all energies[3]	1
Neutrons, energy < 10 keV	5
10 keV to 100 keV	10
> 100 keV to 2 MeV	20
> 2 MeV to 20 MeV	10
> 20 MeV	5
(See also Figure 1)	
Protons, other than recoil protons, energy > 2 MeV	5
Alpha particles, fission fragments, heavy nuclei	20

[1] All values relate to the radiation incident on the body or, for internal sources, emitted from the source.

[2] The choice of values for other radiations is discussed in Annex A.

[3] Excluding Auger electrons emitted from nuclei bound to DNA (see paragraph 26).

Table S-2. Tissue weighting factors[1]

Tissue or organ	Tissue weighting factor, w_T
Gonads	0.20
Bone marrow (red)	0.12
Colon	0.12
Lung	0.12
Stomach	0.12
Bladder	0.05
Breast	0.05
Liver	0.05
Oesophagus	0.05
Thyroid	0.05
Skin	0.01
Bone surface	0.01
Remainder	0.05[2,3]

[1] The values have been developed from a reference population of equal numbers of both sexes and a wide range of ages. In the definition of effective dose they apply to workers, to the whole population, and to either sex.

[2] For purposes of calculation, the remainder is composed of the following additional tissues and organs: adrenals, brain, upper large intestine, small intestine, kidney, muscle, pancreas, spleen, thymus and uterus. The list includes organs which are likely to be selectively irradiated. Some organs in the list are known to be susceptible to cancer induction. If other tissues and organs subsequently become identified as having a significant risk of induced cancer they will then be included either with a specific w_T or in this additional list constituting the remainder. The latter may also include other tissues or organs selectively irradiated.

[3] In those exceptional cases in which a single one of the remainder tissues or organs receives an equivalent dose in excess of the highest dose in any of the twelve organs for which a weighting factor is specified, a weighting factor of 0.025 should be applied to that tissue or organ and a weighting factor of 0.025 to the average dose in the rest of the remainder as defined above.

(S6) Deterministic effects result from the killing of cells which, if the dose is large enough, causes sufficient cell loss to impair the function of the tissue. The probability of causing such harm will be zero at small doses, but above some level of dose (the threshold for clinical effect) the probability will increase steeply to unity (100%). Above the threshold, the severity of the harm will increase with dose. Thresholds for these effects are often at doses of a few Gy or dose rates of a fraction of a Gy per year.

(S7) An important observation in children exposed in utero during a critical 8–15 week period, at Hiroshima and Nagasaki, is a downward shift in the distribution of IQ with increasing dose which can result, after higher doses, in an increase in the probability of severe mental retardation. The effect is presumed to be deterministic with a threshold related to the minimum shift in IQ that can be recognised.

(S8) Stochastic effects may result when an irradiated cell is modified rather than killed. Modified somatic cells may subsequently, after a prolonged delay, develop into a cancer. There are repair and defence mechanisms that make this a very improbable outcome. Nevertheless, the probability of a cancer resulting from radiation increases with increments of dose, probably with no threshold. The severity of the cancer is not affected by the dose. If the damage occurs in a cell whose function is to transmit genetic information to later generations, any resulting effects, which may be of many different kinds and severity, are expressed in the progeny of the exposed person. This type of stochastic effect is called "hereditary".

(S9) The Commission has estimated the probability of a fatal cancer by relying mainly on studies of the Japanese survivors of the atomic bombs and their assessment by bodies such as UNSCEAR and BEIR. These committees have estimated the lifetime cancer risk by considering the accumulated data to 1985, the new dosimetry (DS86) and projection to lifetime by a multiplicative or modified multiplicative model, for high dose, high dose rate exposure. The Commission has concluded, after reviewing the available experimental information on dose–response relationships and the influence of dose and dose rate, that the most probable response is linear quadratic in form for low LET radiation. The linear coefficient at low doses or low dose rates is obtained from the high dose, high dose rate estimates of risk by dividing by a DDREF (dose and dose rate effectiveness factor) of 2. The nominal fatal cancer probabilities for a working population and for a general population, which differ somewhat because of the greater sensitivity of young people, are given in Table S-3. The Commission has made its own estimates of how this fatal cancer risk is distributed among organs and the length of life lost for cancer in each of these organs, by further analysis of the data on the atomic bomb survivors.

(S10) The estimates of severe hereditary effects are also based on the assessments of UNSCEAR and BEIR of experimental data on genetic effects in animals. Evidence suggests that these estimates are not less than the corresponding effects in man. For low dose and dose rates, the probability coefficient for severe hereditary effects in all generations (resulting about equally from dominant and X-linked mutations on the one hand, and multifactorial diseases weighted for severity on the other) are given for both a working population and a general population in Table S-3.

(S11) The Commission uses the term detriment to represent the combination of the probability of occurrence of a harmful health effect and a judgement of the severity of that effect. The many aspects of detriment make it undesirable to select a single quantity to represent the detriment and the Commission has therefore adopted a multi-dimensional concept. The principal components of detriment are the following stochastic quantities: the probability of attributable fatal cancer, the weighted probability of

Table S-3. Nominal probability coefficients for stochastic effects

| Exposed population | Detriment $(10^{-2} \, Sv^{-1})$[1] | | | |
	Fatal cancer[2]	Non-fatal cancer	Severe hereditary effects	Total
Adult workers	4.0	0.8	0.8	5.6
Whole population	5.0	1.0	1.3	7.3

[1] Rounded values.
[2] For fatal cancer, the detriment is equal to the probability coefficient.

attributable non-fatal cancer, the weighted probability of severe hereditary effects and the length of life lost if the harm occurs. The values of this aggregated detriment at low dose for both a working population and a general population are also given in Table S-3.

(S12) The Commission has also assessed the distribution of the detriment in organs and tissues by considering first the fatal cancer probability in each of them, multiplying by an appropriate factor for non-fatal cancer (which is determined by the severity (lethality factor) for that cancer), adding in the probability of severe hereditary effects and adjusting for the relative length of life lost. This distribution of aggregate detriment among organs is represented, after appropriate rounding, by the tissue weighting factors, w_T, given in Table S-2.

(S13) The effective dose is the sum of the weighted equivalent doses in all the tissues and organs of the body. It is given by the expression

$$E = \sum_T w_T \cdot H_T$$

where H_T is the equivalent dose in tissue or organ T and w_T is the weighting factor for tissue T. The effective dose can also be expressed as the sum of the doubly weighted absorbed dose in all the tissues and organs of the body.

The Conceptual Framework of Radiological Protection

(S14) A system of radiological protection should aim to do more good than harm, should call for protection arrangements that maximise the net benefit, and should aim to limit the inequity that may arise from a conflict of interest between individuals and society as a whole.

(S15) Some human activities increase the overall exposure to radiation. The Commission calls these human activities "practices". Other human activities can decrease the overall exposure by influencing the existing causes of exposure. The Commission describes these activities as "intervention".

(S16) The Commission uses a division into three types of exposure: occupational exposure, which is the exposure incurred at work, and principally as a result of work; medical exposure, which is principally the exposure of persons as part of their diagnosis or treatment; and public exposure, which comprises all other exposures.

(S17) In practices and in intervention, it will often be virtually certain that exposures will occur and their magnitude will be predictable, albeit with some degree of error. Sometimes, however, there will be a potential for exposure, but no certainty that it will occur. The Commission calls such exposures "potential exposures".

The system of protection in practices

(S18) The system of radiological protection recommended by the Commission for proposed and continuing practices is based on the following general principles.

(a) No practice involving exposures to radiation should be adopted unless it produces sufficient benefit to the exposed individuals or to society to offset the radiation detriment it causes. (The justification of a practice.)

(b) In relation to any particular source within a practice, the magnitude of individual doses, the number of people exposed, and the likelihood of incurring exposures where these are not certain to be received should all be kept as low as reasonably achievable, economic and social factors being taken into account. This procedure should be constrained by restrictions on the doses to individuals (dose constraints), or the risks to individuals in the case of potential exposures (risk constraints), so as to limit the inequity likely to result from the inherent economic and social judgements. (The optimisation of protection.)

(c) The exposure of individuals resulting from the combination of all the relevant practices should be subject to dose limits, or to some control of risk in the case of potential exposures. These are aimed at ensuring that no individual is exposed to radiation risks that are judged to be unacceptable from these practices in any normal circumstances. Not all sources are susceptible of control by action at the source and it is necessary to specify the sources to be included as relevant before selecting a dose limit. (Individual dose and risk limits.)

The system of protection in intervention

(S19) The system of radiological protection recommended by the Commission for intervention is based on the following general principles.

(a) The proposed intervention should do more good than harm, i.e. the reduction in detriment resulting from the reduction in dose should be sufficient to justify the harm and the costs, including social costs, of the intervention.

(b) The form, scale, and duration of the intervention should be optimised so that the net benefit of the reduction of dose, i.e. the benefit of the reduction in radiation detriment, less the detriment associated with the intervention, should be maximised.

Dose limits do not apply in the case of intervention. Principles (a) and (b) can lead to intervention levels which give guidance to the situations in which intervention is appropriate. There will be some level of projected dose above which, because of serious deterministic effects, intervention will almost always be justified.

(S20) Any system of protection should include an overall assessment of its effectiveness in practice. This should be based on the distribution of doses achieved and on an appraisal of the steps taken to limit the probability of potential exposures. It is important that the basic principles should be treated as a coherent system. No one part should be taken in isolation.

The Control of Occupational Exposure

Dose constraints

(S21) An important feature of optimisation is the choice of dose constraints, the source-related values of individual dose used to limit the range of options considered in the procedure of optimisation. For many types of occupation, it is possible to reach conclusions about the level of individual doses likely to be incurred in well-managed operations. This information can then be used to establish a dose constraint for that type of occupation. The class of occupation should be specified in fairly broad terms, such as work in x-ray diagnostic departments, the routine operation of nuclear plant, or the inspection and maintenance of nuclear plant. Limits prescribed by regulatory agencies and restrictions applied by managements to specific operations as part of the day-to-day control of exposures are not constraints in the sense used here. In general, they should be established on the basis of the results of optimisation. It will usually be appropriate for dose constraints to be fixed at the national or local level.

Dose limits

(S22) The dose limits for application in occupational exposure are summarised in Table S-4.

(S23) Dose limits are needed as part of the control of occupational exposure, both to impose a limit on the choice of dose constraints and to provide a protection against errors of judgement in the application of optimisation.

(S24) In setting dose limits, the Commission's aim is to establish, for a defined set of practices, and for regular and continued exposure, a level of dose above which the consequences for the individual would be widely regarded as unacceptable. In the past, the Commission has used the attributable probability of death or severe hereditary disorders as the basis for judging the consequences of an exposure. This quantity is still a major factor, but is no longer regarded by the Commission as sufficient to describe the detriment.

(S25) The Commission recommends a limit on effective dose of 20 mSv per year, averaged over 5 years (100 mSv in 5 years), with the further provision that the effective

Table S-4. Recommended dose limits[1]

| Application | Dose limit | |
	Occupational	Public
Effective dose	20 mSv per year, averaged over defined periods of 5 years[2]	1 mSv in a year[3]
Annual equivalent dose in		
the lens of the eye	150 mSv	15 mSv
the skin[4]	500 mSv	50 mSv
the hands and feet	500 mSv	—

[1] The limits apply to the sum of the relevant doses from external exposure in the specified period and the 50-year committed dose (to age 70 years for children) from intakes in the same period (see paragraph 143).

[2] With the further provision that the effective dose should not exceed 50 mSv in any single year. Additional restrictions apply to the occupational exposure of pregnant women, which is discussed in Section 5.3.3 of the Main Text.

[3] In special circumstances, a higher value of effective dose could be allowed in a single year, provided that the average over 5 years does not exceed 1 mSv per year.

[4] The limitation on the effective dose provides sufficient protection for the skin against stochastic effects. An additional limit is needed for localised exposures in order to prevent deterministic effects. (See paragraphs 173 and 194.)

dose should not exceed 50 mSv in any single year. The 5-year period would have to be defined by the regulatory agency, e.g. as discrete 5-year calendar periods. The Commission would not expect the period to be introduced and then applied retrospectively. It is implicit in these recommended dose limits that the dose constraint for optimisation should not exceed 20 mSv in a year.

(S26) Subject to medical advice in individual cases, there need be no special restrictions applied to the exposure of an individual following a control period in which the exposure of the individual has exceeded a dose limit. Such events should call for a thorough examination, usually by the regulatory agency, of the design and operational aspects of protection in the installation concerned, rather than for restrictions or penalties applied to the exposed individual. If the dose is unknown, or is thought to be high, referral to a physician should be considered.

(S27) The recommended limits should apply to all forms of occupational exposure, unless special provisions have been made by the regulatory agency. Because of the difficulties of responding rapidly to an increase in stringency in operations on plant and equipment already in existence, the Commission recognises that regulatory agencies may wish to make temporary use of higher dose limits. Such arrangements should be regarded as transient.

(S28) The dose limit forms only a part of the system of protection aimed at achieving levels of dose that are as low as reasonably achievable, economic and social factors being taken into account. It is not to be seen as a target. It represents, in the Commission's view, the point at which regular, extended, deliberate, occupational exposure can reasonably be regarded as only just tolerable.

(S29) The restrictions on effective dose are sufficient to ensure the avoidance of deterministic effects in all body tissues and organs except the lens of the eye, which makes a negligible contribution to the effective dose, and the skin, which may well be subject to localised exposures. Separate dose limits are needed for these tissues. The annual limits are 150 mSv for the lens and 500 mSv for the skin, averaged over any 1 cm², regardless of the area exposed.

(S30) For internal exposure, annual limits on intake will be based on a committed effective dose of 20 mSv. The estimated intakes may be averaged over a period of 5 years to provide some flexibility. The occupational limits for radon are under review. Meanwhile, the values given in *Publication 47* (1986) remain valid.

The occupational exposure of women

(S31) The basis for the control of the occupational exposure of women who are not pregnant is the same as that for men and the Commission recommends no special occupational dose limit for women in general.

(S32) Once pregnancy has been declared, the conceptus should be protected by applying a supplementary equivalent dose limit to the surface of the woman's abdomen (lower trunk) of 2 mSv for the remainder of the pregnancy and by limiting intakes of radionuclides to about 1/20 of the ALI. The Commission wishes to emphasise that the use of its system of protection, particularly the use of source-related dose constraints, will usually provide an adequate guarantee of compliance with this limit without the need for specific restrictions on the employment of pregnant women. The principal criterion will then be that the employment should be of a type that does not carry a significant probability of high accidental doses and intakes. High-dose and high-risk occupations from which pregnant women should be excluded should be defined by regulatory agencies.

The Control of Medical Exposure

(S33) In the justification of a practice leading to medical exposures, the practice should be defined in broad terms. However, each procedure, either diagnostic or therapeutic, is subject to a separate decision, so that there is an opportunity to apply a further, case-by-case, justification for each procedure. This will not be necessary for simple diagnostic procedures based on common indications, but may be important for complex investigations and for therapy.

(S34) There is considerable scope for dose reductions in diagnostic radiology using the techniques of optimisation of protection. Consideration should be given to the use of dose constraints, or investigation levels, selected by the appropriate professional or regulatory agency, for application in some common diagnostic procedures. They should be applied with flexibility to allow higher doses where indicated by sound clinical judgement.

(S35) Constraints should also be considered in the optimisation of protection for medical exposures when the procedures are not intended to be of direct value to the exposed individual, as in scientific and clinical studies involving the exposure of volunteers.

(S36) Medical exposures are usually intended to provide a direct benefit to the exposed individual. If the practice is justified and the protection optimised, the dose in the patient will be as low as is compatible with the medical purposes. The Commission therefore recommends that dose limits should not be applied to medical exposures. Further, it is not appropriate to include the doses incurred by patients in the course of diagnostic examinations or therapy when considering compliance with dose limits applied to occupational or public exposures.

(S37) Diagnostic and therapeutic procedures causing exposures of the abdomen of women likely to be pregnant should be avoided unless there are strong clinical indications. Information on possible pregnancy should be obtained from the patient herself. If the most recent expected menstruation has been missed, and there is no other relevant information, the woman should be assumed to be pregnant.

The Control of Public Exposure

(S38) The control of public exposure in all normal situations is exercised by the application of controls at the source rather than in the environment. The controls are achieved almost entirely by the procedures of constrained optimisation and the use of prescriptive limits. It is often convenient to class together individuals who form a homogeneous group with respect to their exposures to a single source. When such a group is typical of those most highly exposed by that source, it is known as a critical group. The dose constraint should be applied to the mean dose in the critical group from the source for which the protection is being optimised.

Dose limits

(S39) The scope of dose limits for public exposure is confined to the doses incurred as the result of practices. Doses incurred in situations where the only available protective action takes the form of intervention are excluded from that scope. Separate attention has to be paid to potential exposures. Radon in dwellings and in the open air, radioactive materials, natural or artificial, already in the environment, and other natural sources are examples of situations that can be influenced only by intervention. Doses from these sources are therefore outside the scope of the dose limits for public exposure. The conduct of intervention involves occupational exposure and should be treated accordingly.

(S40) The Commission now recommends that the limit for public exposure should be expressed as an effective dose of 1 mSv in a year. However, in special circumstances, a higher value of effective dose could be allowed in a single year, provided that the average over 5 years does not exceed 1 mSv per year.

(S41) In selecting the limit on effective dose, the Commission has sought a value that would be only just short of unacceptable for continued exposure as the result of deliberate practices the use of which is a matter of choice. This does not imply that higher doses from other sources, such as radon in dwellings, should be regarded as unacceptable. The existence of these sources may be undesirable but is not a matter of choice. The doses can be controlled only by intervention, which will also have undesirable features.

(S42) Limits are also needed for the lens of the eye and skin since these tissues will not necessarily be protected against deterministic effects by the limit on effective dose. The Commission recommends annual limits of 15 mSv for the lens and 50 mSv for the skin averaged over any 1 cm^2, regardless of the area exposed. The recommended limits are summarised in Table S-4.

Potential Exposures

(S43) The initial treatment of potential exposures should form part of the system of protection applied to practices, but it should be recognised that the exposures, if they occur, may lead to intervention. At this stage, there should be two objectives, prevention and mitigation. Prevention is the reduction of the probability of the sequences of events that may cause or increase radiation exposures. Mitigation is the limitation and reduction of the exposures if any of these sequences do occur. A great deal can be accomplished at the stages of design and operation to reduce the consequences of accident sequences so that intervention may not become necessary.

(S44) In order to maintain a strict coherence in the treatment of actual and potential exposures, it would be necessary to extend the concept of detriment to include the probability of occurrence of the situation giving rise to the detriment. Techniques for achieving this are still being developed. A comprehensive approach to this problem calls for the application of multi-attribute analysis.

(S45) A simpler approach is possible for both individual and collective exposures if the doses will be small even if the event occurs. If the doses, should they occur, will not be in excess of dose limits, it is adequate to use the product of the expected dose and its probability of occurrence as if this were a dose that was certain to occur. The conventional procedures of justification and optimisation can then be applied.

The System of Protection in Intervention

(S46) Before a programme of intervention is initiated, it should be demonstrated that the proposed intervention will be justified, i.e. do more good than harm, and that the form, scale, and duration of the intervention have been chosen so as to optimise the protection. The processes of justification and optimisation both apply to the protective action, so it is necessary to consider them together when reaching a decision. Justification is the process of deciding that the disadvantages of each component of intervention, i.e. of each protective action, are more than offset by the reductions in the dose likely to be achieved. Optimisation is the process of deciding on the method, scale and duration of the action so as to obtain the maximum net benefit. In simple terms, the difference between the disadvantages and the benefits, expressed in the same terms, e.g. costs, including social costs with an allowance for anxiety, should be positive for each protective action adopted and should be maximised by settling the details of that action.

Radon in Dwellings

(S47) Radon in dwellings needs special attention because both the individual and the collective doses from radon are higher than those from almost any other source. If improvements are needed in existing dwellings, they have to be achieved by intervention involving modifications to the dwellings or to the behaviour of the occupants.

(S48) The Commission recommended the use of action levels to help in deciding when to require or advise remedial action in existing dwellings. The choice of an action level is complex, depending not only on the level of exposure, but also on the likely scale of action, which has economic implications for the community and for individuals. For new dwellings, guides or codes for their construction in selected areas can be established so that it is highly probable that exposures in these dwellings will be below some chosen reference level. The Commission has initiated a further review of current experience with a view to issuing revised recommendations in due course. Meanwhile the guidance in *Publication 39* (1984) should still be used.

Intervention After Accidents

(S49) The benefit of a particular protective action within a programme of intervention should be judged on the basis of the reduction in dose achieved or expected by that specific protective action, i.e. the dose averted. Thus each protective action has to be considered on its own merits. In addition, however, the doses that would be incurred via all the relevant pathways of exposure, some subject to protective actions and some not, should be assessed. If the total dose in some individuals is so high as to be unacceptable even in an emergency, the feasibility of additional protective actions influencing the major contributions to the total dose should be urgently reviewed. Doses causing serious deterministic effects or a high probability of stochastic effects would call for such a review.

(S50) Occupational exposures of emergency teams during emergency and remedial action can be limited by operational controls. Some relaxation of the controls for normal situations can be permitted in serious accidents without lowering the long-term level of protection. This relaxation should not permit the exposures in the control of the accident and in the immediate and urgent remedial work to give effective doses of more than about 0.5 Sv except for life-saving actions, which can rarely be limited by dosimetric assessments. The equivalent dose to skin should not be allowed to exceed about 5 Sv. Once the immediate emergency is under control, remedial work should be treated as part of the occupational exposure incurred in a practice.

Practical Implementation of the Commission's Recommendations

(S51) Chapter 7 of the recommendations emphasises the importance of the operational level of radiological protection and shows how this should be developed from the requirements of regulatory agencies and the recommendations of the Commission. The Commission now recommends that the designation of controlled and supervised areas should be decided either at the design stage or locally by the operating management on the basis of operational experience and judgement. The classification of working conditions based upon expected dose is no longer recommended. The Chapter gives advice on the measurement of doses (monitoring and record keeping) and on medical surveillance. It also discusses emergency planning and the bases for exemption from regulatory requirements. It deals with both practices and intervention.

SUBJECT INDEX

Individual items in this edition are indexed by paragraph number.

Annals of the ICRP

Aims and Scope

Founded in 1928, the International Commission on Radiological Protection has, since 1950, been providing general guidance on the widespread use of radiation sources caused by developments in the field of nuclear energy.

The reports and recommendations of the ICRP are available in the form of a review journal, *Annals of the ICRP*. Subscribers to the journal will receive each new report as soon as it appears, thus ensuring that they are kept abreast of the latest developments in this important field, and can build up a complete set of ICRP reports and recommendations.

Single issues of the journal are available separately for those individuals and organizations who do not require a complete set of all ICRP publications, but would like to have their own copy of a particular report covering their own field of interest. Please order through your bookseller, subscription agent or, in case of difficulty, direct from the publisher.

Publications of the ICRP
Full details of all ICRP reports can be obtained from your nearest Pergamon Press office.

Published reports of the ICRP

(Continued)